MW01482176

Great Sex

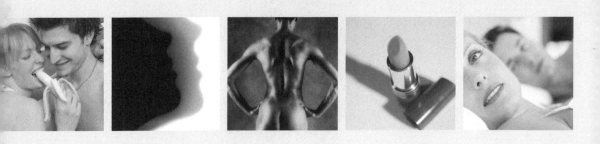

52 Brilliant Ideas

one good idea can change your life

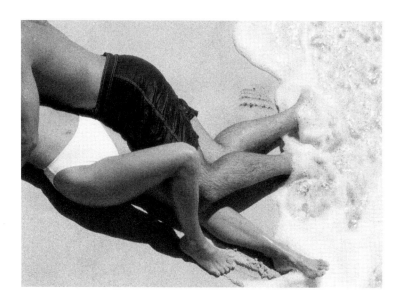

Great Sex

Bigger, Better, Faster, More

Elisabeth Wilson

A Perigee Book

A PERIGEE BOOK
Published by the Penguin Group
Penguin Group (USA) Inc.
375 Hudson Street, New York, New York 10014, USA
Penguin Group (Canada), 90 Eglinton Avenue East, Suite 700, Toronto, Ontario M4P 2Y3, Canada
(a division of Pearson Penguin Canada Inc.)
Penguin Books Ltd., 80 Strand, London WC2R 0RL, England
Penguin Group Ireland, 25 St. Stephen's Green, Dublin 2, Ireland (a division of Penguin Books Ltd.)
Penguin Group (Australia), 250 Camberwell Road, Camberwell, Victoria 3124, Australia
(a division of Pearson Australia Group Pty. Ltd.)
Penguin Books India Pvt. Ltd., 11 Community Centre, Panchsheel Park, New Delhi—110 017, India
Penguin Group (NZ), 67 Apollo Drive, Rosedale, North Shore 0632, New Zealand
(a division of Pearson New Zealand Ltd.)
Penguin Books (South Africa) (Pty.) Ltd., 24 Sturdee Avenue, Rosebank, Johannesburg 2196,
South Africa

Penguin Books Ltd., Registered Offices: 80 Strand, London WC2R 0RL, England

While the author has made every effort to provide accurate telephone numbers and Internet addresses at the time of publication, neither the publisher nor the author assumes any responsibility for errors, or for changes that occur after publication. Further, the publisher does not have any control over and does not assume any responsibility for author or third-party websites or their content.

GREAT SEX

Copyright © 2005 by The Infinite Ideas Company Limited
Cover design by Liz Sheehan
Text design by Baseline Arts Ltd., Oxford

All rights reserved.
No part of this book may be reproduced, scanned, or distributed in any printed or electronic form without permission. Please do not participate in or encourage piracy of copyrighted materials in violation of the author's rights. Purchase only authorized editions.
PERIGEE is a registered trademark of Penguin Group (USA) Inc.
The "P" design is a trademark belonging to Penguin Group (USA) Inc.

First American edition: February 2008
Originally published as *Re-energise Your Sex Life* in Great Britain in 2005 by The Infinite Ideas Company Limited.

Perigee trade paperback ISBN: 978-0-399-53392-1

PRINTED IN THE UNITED STATES OF AMERICA

10   9   8   7   6   5   4   3   2   1

Most Perigee books are available at special quantity discounts for bulk purchases for sales promotions, premiums, fund-raising, or educational use. Special books, or book excerpts, can also be created to fit specific needs. For details, write: Special Markets, Penguin Group (USA) Inc., 375 Hudson Street, New York, New York 10014.

Brilliant ideas

Brilliant features

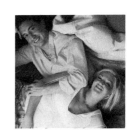

Each chapter of this book is designed to provide you with an inspirational idea that you can read quickly and put into practice right away.

Throughout you'll find four features that will help you to get straight to the heart of the idea:

- *Try another idea* If this idea looks like a life-changer then there's no time to lose. *Try another idea* will point you right to a related tip to expand and enhance the first.

- *Here's an idea for you* Give it a try—right here, right now—and get an idea of how well you're doing so far.

- *Defining ideas* Words of wisdom from masters and mistresses of the art, plus some interesting hangers-on.

- *How did it go?* If at first you do succeed, try to hide your amazement. If, on the other hand, you don't, this is where you'll find a Q and A that highlights common problems and how to get over them.

Introduction

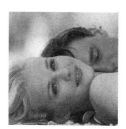

We promise you no crummy line drawings of silly positions, no step-by-step instructions on starting your own bisexual swinging club, and no illustrations of bearded hippie guys looking masterful.

We've kept those promises. You'll have read everything in this book before and we don't pretend otherwise. In fact, we're proud of that. Because the success of a book promising to transform your sex life doesn't lie in its risqué content or its lack of it. A sex book will only work if it's doable. Readers should want to act on the suggestions rather than just read them for vicarious thrills or, more likely, in growing consternation.

This is a book of sex solutions, not potential problems. So there's nothing in here about safe sex. If you're young, free, and single, desperate to mingle and push your sexual boundaries, then this book is not for you. Continue with the group sex in tents at Burning Man, people. We salute you, but we've been there, done that, and we'd rather stay beneath our duvets. This book is for couples who simply want to have better sex with the person they're with. And they've probably been with that person for quite a long time. (Also, although this information is broadly aimed at heterosexual couples, I hope gay and lesbian couples find their interests well-served, too.)

What these people want (and I include myself here) are quick, reliable, and above all easy ways to reignite the fire. We don't want this to involve expensive props, embarrassing encounters, vinyl nurse's outfits, or to interfere with our soap opera habit. And that's where this book comes into its own. I decided to write it because I believe that the 52 ideas format is the best possible way to encourage people not simply to read but to experience. Because of my work, I've read more sex books than most other people have had orgasms and I know that for sex advice to work you have to actually act upon it rather than simply read it. So, all of the ideas have been tested by real couples (thanks, and I promise not to reveal your names). The very simplest ideas can have you feeling new sensations or rediscovering old favorites, as I found out after undertaking my very first piece of "research" involving nothing more than a bottle of vodka (see IDEA 24). As we all know, but tend to forget, the basis of great sex over the long-term is that old chestnut, communication. And I discovered that it doesn't take a lot to get you talking to each other again about what you like and what you don't. At the very least, these ideas can give you a great laugh when they go wrong and can blow your socks off when they go right.

Sex in most long-term relationships isn't the most important component, but my own feeling is that if more of us were to give it a much higher priority we'd be a lot happier. To quote Erica Jong, "There are things that happen in the dark between two people that make everything that happens in the light all right." For very little effort, you can improve your sex life greatly. It says 52 ideas on the cover of this book but in my persnickety way, I've counted them and there are actually 403. If you and your partner try just ten of these over the next twelve months (much less ten weeks), you'll improve your love life beyond recognition. That's more than you can say about line drawings of the "split bamboo" position.

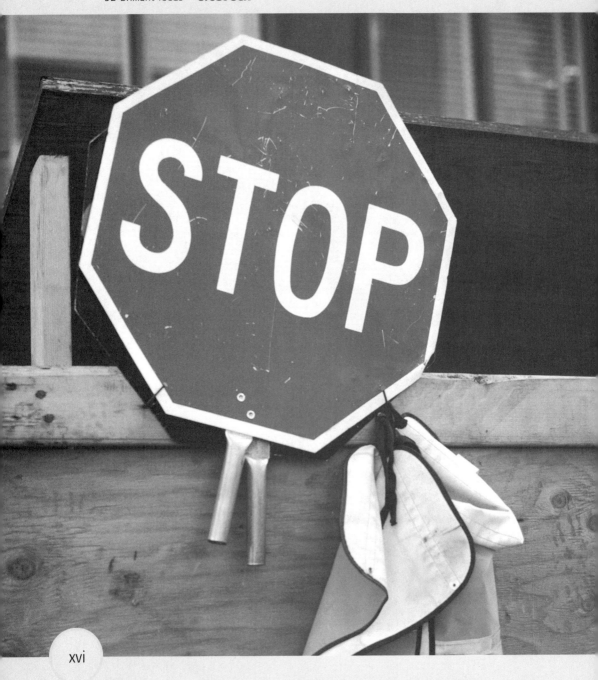

1

Stop having sex

Bored with sex? Then take a break.

Focusing on sensuality rather than sex can remind you why sex is worth bothering with in the first place.

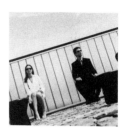

The top tool in the sexual counseling box of tricks is a technique called "sensate focus." To put it bluntly, you make a pact not to have penetrative sex. When couples go to see a sex therapist, they will often be asked to refrain until they've worked through their "issues." Couples will often spend weeks simply holding each other, working up to touching each other non-sexually through techniques such as massage, and then finally moving on to sexual pleasuring without penetrative sex. If you got stuck at the beginning of the last sentence, focusing on the word "weeks" with a sort of sick dread, then relax. You don't have to give up sex for all that long to get astounding results.

Giving up sex completely sounds extreme, but couples find that taking a break from disappointed expectations and performance pressure—and instead spending time getting to know each other again through strictly non-penetrative contact—works wonders when they want to regain their passion. Ripping apart old patterns of

Here's an idea for you... **Don't focus on the outcome. Don't consciously try to arouse your partner. Concentrate only on touch. The person being touched should try to dissolve into it and concentrate on the sensations. This is a sort of meditation for both of you and should at the very least help you to relax when you're frazzled.**

relating to each other means couples get back to basics. Simply spending time with each other trying to make your partner feel good is powerful. You'll remember what all the fuss was about in the first place.

Sex expert Tracey Cox says sex is like chocolate— if we get too much of a good thing we get sick of it. Think how much better chocolate tastes after you've given it up for Lent. It's the same thing with sex. Too much and we get jaded and take it for granted.

You might be far from needing sex therapy, but there are very few couples who wouldn't benefit from a little sensate focus. It encourages better communication and sparks libido.

Choose a week when you both decide that you won't have penetrative sex.

Day 1   On the first night you cuddle up together on the couch.

Day 2   Go to bed an hour early. Naked. Lie in bed stroking and touching each other. Talk about your lives. Reconnect.

Day 3   Take a shower or bath together with sensual oils.

Day 4 She gives him a long all-over massage.

Day 5 He gives her a long all-over massage.

Day 6 She massages him, including touching him sexually but not to the point where he has an orgasm. She can explore his reactions to various kinds of touching and ask for feedback.

Day 7 He does the same for her.

Day 8 By now the sexual tension between you should be causing visible sparks!

Try sensate focus in your bathroom to give a whole new meaning to good, clean fun. Look at IDEA 34, *The love bath*.

Try another idea...

"He was the kind of guy who could kiss you behind your ear and make you feel like you'd just had kinky sex."
JULIA ALVAREZ, writer

Defining idea...

3

How was
it for
you?

Q   We don't have a clear week to devote to this. Any ideas?

A   *Try some speed sensate focus. It's like speed dating, but less embarrassing.
Use a little sensory deprivation to help you focus on the power of touch.
It's a great reminder when we're tired and wired that our bodies can give
us supreme physical pleasure. The more senses that are cut off, the more
we appreciate the ones that are left. Blindfold your partner and then insist
they relax totally for the next fifteen minutes. They could wear earplugs,
too, to really sink into their own world of sensory delight. Play some soft
music for your benefit and light some candles. Ask your partner to lie back
on comfortable pillows or a duvet. They should be naked and you should
either be lightly dressed or naked. The room should be warm. Using a long
feather or a soft silk scarf, stroke every part of your partner's body, not just
the usual erogenous zones. Keep the touch gentle and continuous. Finally,
blow gently over their skin everywhere the feather or silk touched. You can
then switch places.*

Q   What if I'm just not comfortable with all that touchy-feely stuff?

A   *Ignore your need for sensuality—and that of your partner's—at your peril.
The need to be held lovingly is fundamental to humans. Scientists believe it
could be as important in our behavioral development as food and water. We
crave sensual touch and for many of us sex is the means whereby we get it.
Orgasm could simply be the payoff that nature's built into our physiological
makeup to make sure we seek out physical closeness—especially where
women are concerned, since orgasm isn't strictly necessary for reproduction.*

2

Getting it right

How do you get your lover to love you the way you want to be loved?

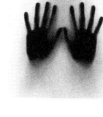

Just because you've been together forever doesn't mean you press each other's buttons absolutely perfectly. Yet the man or woman who can tell their lover that they want to be touched differently from the way they've been touched a million times before is pretty rare.

There are ways to ask without embarrassing yourself and mortifying your lover. Here's how to get your lover to do something differently when they think they've been getting it right for years.

Here's an idea for you...
Always find something positive to say, but don't praise what's bad. Pretending to enjoy what you don't enjoy is what got you in this mess in the first place!

THE WRONG WAY

Using phrases starting with "Why don't you…," "You never…," or "That doesn't…" will cause offense and your partner will get defensive. Moreover, whining is deeply unattractive.

THE RIGHT WAY

Step 1: Praise, praise, praise—your new resolution

From now on, you're going to be an appreciative lover. You're going to praise your lover's performance every chance you get and using every way you can think of. This will create a "win–win" situation. Be especially appreciative during sex. Do it with body language. Do it loudly. Spell it out: "I love everything you do in bed," "You're just so sexy," "No one's ever done that to me the way that you do." They should finish every session assured that you're blissfully happy.

If you're not an appreciative lover, make this your modus operandi from now on. For one thing, this technique will backfire spectacularly on you if it stops as soon as you get what you want—it will look like a cynical ploy. (That's because it *will* be a cynical ploy.) So wise up: There's nothing to be ashamed of in creating confidence in your lover. Their "win" is that you're creating an atmosphere where they can't fail. They won't fear trying something different if they don't feel that your happiness is dependent on it. If they get it wrong or if they don't want to go through with it, they've got nothing to lose because they know just how much you value them. Your "win" is that besides being a lovely person you're also gearing them up for moving your sex life on to greater heights.

Step 2: Focus on the positive

Once you've created a climate of confidence, you can modify their technique by focusing on the positive. For instance, "I love the way you do that, especially when you go slowly/quickly/hang off the bedside table while you're doing it." The other great bonus of this approach is that, within reason, it doesn't matter if it's a complete lie. For example, your lover may fellate you with the speed of a jackhammer, but if you tell her how lovely it is when her mouth goes really slowly she'll probably believe you. She'll almost certainly start doing it slowly, too. The payoff for you is that you'll get more of what you want.

This clearly can be overdone. She's obviously going to get suspicious if she never hangs off the edge of the bedside table while doing it yet you can't stop talking it up. Use discretion and be specific if possible. And you really need to use your hands to gently direct the action the way you want it.

Step 3: Suggest how they could change

Now you can suggest doing it differently. This has to be done with grace and it has to be done lightly, not as if your entire sexual happiness depends on it (remember, they can't fail). Say that you've read about something you'd like to try in a book and ask if they would give it a shot…

See IDEA 17, *Learn the art of kaizen,* **and get more of what you want.**

Try another idea…

"The secret to telling someone they're the worst lover you've ever had, is…not to. Focus on what you want, not what you don't…Start by focusing on yourself, not your partner's [faults]. Make a list of ten things you want more of in bed, ten things you want less of, and ten new things you'd like to try. You have to know what you want in bed in order to get it."
TRACEY COX, *Supersex*

Defining idea…

7

Q   **I tried this but my lover is very self-conscious. Any other ideas?**

A   *Some couples find it helps to use the virgin fantasy when they're trying something new. Another version is the alien fantasy. Basically, one of you is a virgin/alien and has no idea what sex is. The other person has to explain what they should do, how they should behave, and what they should say. This works well because the shier, more self-conscious person isn't in control—they're only following instructions.*

Q   **His oral sex technique has improved a lot, but it's still not hitting the right buttons. What now?**

A   *If your communication is good then you're just going to have to show him. Make it during a very steamy session where you're both a bit crazed with passion and he wants to do anything to get you off. Ask him, "Would you mind trying this? I've been thinking it would really drive me crazy." Then show him with your own tongue, on his bicep, palm, or any other flat surface (men can do this on a woman's finger or toes). Make sure he can see what your tongue is doing and how fast it's going. Back this up with instructions, but only a little at a time. Aim for a 10 percent improvement every time. And praise, praise, praise.*

3

Lust—it's all in your mind

Not as interested as you used to be? The easiest way out of a rut is to get sex on the brain—literally.

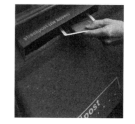

Researching this book has brought up some surprises for me and one of them has been the effect on my own libido.

Always an "average" on the sex-o-meter—in other words, I'm not the girl most likely to suggest a love-in with the neighbors—thinking, reading, and talking about sex for three months has had an extraordinary effect on my sexual response. I don't mean that I've been tempted to give swinging a try, but having sex on the brain has definitely increased my desire for sex and I'll now advise people that the simplest way to ensure you have (and want) more sex is to *think* about it more regularly.

As time goes on, we become subsumed in the minutiae of our lives—the fetching, carrying, hunting, gathering. But as sex writer Ann Hooper says, "You can try every sex position you can think of, including dangling from the ceiling, but if you don't bring your fertile brain into play, you may not manage to become aroused."

The secret is to fantasize. But first you'll have to rethink your idea of what sexual fantasy means.

Here's an idea for you... **Read sexy romance novels or soft porn. Listen to music that makes you feel sexual—whatever it is, if it rocks your boat, play it loud and play it often.**

When did you consistently have the best sex you've ever had? Most of us would say in the first few months of getting it on with a new partner, hopefully the partner we're still with. Why? New love, of course, or new lust at the very least. The principal reason that the sex at the beginning of a relationship is so outstanding is that it's fantasy-fueled. New lovers spend just about every minute they're not in bed with their lover fantasizing about their lover. Their minds are constantly running over what they were doing the night before and what they'd like to be doing next time they meet. They walk around in a fog of erotic fantasy. And this fuels their sexual encounters. The second they see their lover they're primed and ready to go.

We tend to think it's the person that fuels our desperation for sex, but physiologically it's got just as much to do with the mind being constantly focused on doing the deed and the signals this sends to our body. So, if you've wistfully looked back on the way you used to feel about each other and if you firmly believe that you can't reconstruct that lust, try thinking about sex more. Any thoughts you have—no matter how fleeting—count. Think about sex during the day, and when the chance to have sex arrives you're far more likely to be enthusiastic. Just a touch will get the juices flowing. On the other hand, if nary a sexual thought has fluttered across your mind during the day, your lover is going to have an uphill and probably futile struggle to get you to even try.

...and another **Count the number of people you meet in a day who actively appeal to you. Seek to get aroused by other people, but obviously don't act on it. That old chestnut about taking the energy back to stoke the home fires isn't an old chestnut for nothing.**

Counselor Sarah Litvinoff says, "Sex therapists often find that women who claim never to have been sexually interested or who have gone off sex, never think sexual thoughts. Many people narrowly define sexual fantasies as the mini-pornographic scenes you play out in your head, which might include, say, bondage or lesbian images, that are a mental turn-on, but which you wouldn't necessarily enjoy enacting for real. But, in fact, *any* sexual thought is sexual fantasy." And any sort of sexual thought gets the job done.

Turn to IDEA 50, *Dream time*, for more on the power of the mind.

Try another idea...

Let your mind wander, look for the lascivious, and feel the throb of sex that is lying beneath the layers of our sophisticated lifestyle. Find stimulation in your daily routine and you'll find yourself spilling over with erotic charge, which will translate into action. You will initiate sex and respond to your partner in a different way sexually. You'll be begging for it.

Begin to make a habit of daydreaming about sex. First thing when you wake up in the morning or last thing before you go to sleep, think a dirty thought or two. When you're commuting, let the last time you made love run through your mind. As you're waiting for your train, relive your sexual greatest hits. Remember that every time sex flits across your mind it's a fantasy, and that those who fantasize most have the best sex lives.

"You are what you dream. You are what you daydream. Masters and Johnson's charts and numbers and flashing lights and plastic pricks tell us everything about sex and nothing about it. Because sex is all in the head."
ERICA JONG

Defining idea...

Like faith healing, you don't have to believe in this for it to work.

How was
it for
you?

Q   I feel a bit mean fantasizing about anyone but my wife. What can I do?

A   *One woman I know visualizes herself slamming any averagely attractive man she meets against the wall and kissing him wildly. On the surface she's shaking hands and mouthing platitudes. The men know nothing of it, but the sexual frisson created by those images fuels her own idea of her sexual self. Her reasons for doing it have absolutely nothing to do with a desire for infidelity. She says, "It's like being a teenager again. When anyone remotely attractive came into your sights, no matter how 'unsuitable,' you'd start flirting and wondering about a possible liaison, obviously not going anywhere because you were fifteen. Fantasizing like this keeps me young." It's harmless, it's cheap, it's private. But there's no law that says you can't fantasize about your partner in this way if you want. Next time you see a cute waitress, imagine it's your missus bringing you a latte in that low-cut top instead.*

Q   I don't have a sexual thought in my head that vaguely interests me. Where can I begin?

A   *OK, start this way. Imagine yourself being as sexually attractive as you can be. In your mind, you're drop-dead gorgeous. Move on to visualizing this gorgeous you having sex. Stick with this for a while and see what happens.*

4

The least you need to do...

...to keep your relationship minty fresh.

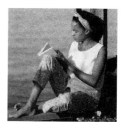

Read, digest, and ponder. Then get your planner, a big red pen, and start prioritizing your relationship.

This chapter contains the three golden rules of a healthy relationship—the sine qua non of sexual happiness. All the technique and creativity in the world isn't going to fix the sex in a relationship where the couple is together but not *together*. On the other hand, couples who spend time together, and anticipate and plan for those times, find it hard to lose interest in each other.

RULE 1: DAILY...

How is your partner feeling right now? What's happening at work? How are their relationships with friends, colleagues, siblings, parents? Carve out fifteen minutes of every day to talk. If you find yourselves getting into a rut of busyness, when you pass like ships in the night for several days in a row without touching base, either go to bed before your usual time or get up earlier and have coffee together so you can catch up.

Here's an idea for you... **Look for easy ways to cheer your partner up. Pick up a tub of her favorite ice cream on the way home from work. Run him a bath and bring him a beer. Sappy gestures work—they build up a huge bank of goodwill that couples can draw on when life gets stressful.**

Kiss each other every morning before you get out of bed. Take the time for a swift cuddle. Breathe deeply. Hold tight. Do the same at night. Never take your physical intimacy for granted. In this Vale of Tears we call life, you found each other. Pretty amazing. Worth acknowledging that with at least a daily hug.

RULE 2: WEEKLY...

Go out with each other once a week whenever humanly possible. Once every two weeks is the bare minimum. According to the experts, this is the most important thing you can do. Couples who keep dating keep mating. Spending too long hanging around the same house does something to a couple's sexual interest in each other and what it does generally isn't good. So get out, preferably after making some small effort to spruce yourself up so you're visually pleasing to your partner. Let them see why they bothered with you in the first place. (No, I never said this chapter was rocket science. I just said that it worked.)

RULE 3: MONTHLY...

Go for a mini-adventure—shared memories cement your relationship. Make your adventure as crazy or calm as you like, but at the least make sure it's something that you haven't done since the beginning of your relationship. It really doesn't matter what it is, as long as it's not your usual "date."

Defining idea... *"Good sex begins when your clothes are still on."*
MASTERS and JOHNSON, sex research pioneers

14

What's the point? You see your partner coping with new environments and new skills and that keeps you interested in them. And them in you. Simple.

The appointment system in IDEA 8, *Sleep is the new sex—honest!*, is a good option if sex has turned into a rushed afterthought.

Try another idea...

If you're shaking your head and tutting "how banal," I'd get that smug look off your face, pronto. Research shows quite clearly that one of the defining differences between strong couples and "drifting" couples is the amount of effort and time they spend on their shared pursuits. All of us have heard the advice, "Spend more time with each other being as interesting as possible." But how many couples do you know who actually do it? I'm prepared to bet that those who do seem happiest.

Q How do you expect us to get out once a week?

A *You don't have to go out for long—an hour or two is fine. Even parents of newborns can find a way if sufficiently motivated.*
No money? Make it a challenge to have a good night out on a tenner or less. If all else fails, go for a walk and treat yourself to a beer at your local bar. Oh OK, share half a beer if money's really tight.
No childcare? Make it your mission to seek out other couples with kids who live locally—ideally, on the next street—and look like they enjoy going out (single parents and confirmed stay-at-homes are no good for this). The deal is that one half of their couple comes to your house and sits with your kids once a week. The next week one of you returns the favor. It means that for one night's babysitting you get two nights out and an evening home alone. Not bad.
No conversation? You'd better fix this one before you do anything else.

How was it for you?

Q **We couldn't come up with anything we wanted to do for a mini-adventure. Any suggestions?**

A *Here's a year's worth:*

- *Hill walking between two cozy inns, restaurants, or bars*
- *Renting bicycles*
- *Al fresco dining, with champagne and strawberries*
- *Horse riding*
- *Paragliding*
- *Spending a weekend in a city you've never visited before*
- *Boating along a river or in your local park*
- *Watching a matinee at the movie theater*
- *Spending a day at a health spa*
- *Visiting an art gallery*
- *Going to the theater*
- *Attending a self-help seminar*

Take turns to suggest the adventure, and go along with your partner's choice even if you aren't that interested initially. Even the disasters will give you shared memories to laugh about afterward.

5

Join the 30 percent

That's the percentage of women who can come purely through penetrative sex. Hmmm.

I think 30 percent is putting it too high. I figure it's nearer to 10 percent. Other surveys report that around 90 percent of women have orgasms only through oral sex or masturbation, and that sounds much closer to the truth.

My point being, most women don't come through penetrative sex. Those of you ladies who do, there's still a big debate over what's rocking your boat. It could be indirect stimulation of the clitoris or rhythmic rubbing of the anterior vaginal wall (home of the elusive G-spot). Anyway, enough about you already.

This chapter is primarily aimed at the majority of women who haven't yet come from straightforward sexual intercourse. There are various ways of making this happen. There are lots of ideas bridging techniques and the G-spot, but here is the lowdown on the one position that's designed to give constant clitoral stimulation during genital intercourse: the coital alignment technique (CAT). A useful one to master because, let's face it, constant clitoral stimulation is no doubt going to up

Here's an idea for you... **Women: Once you've got the hang of the rocking movement squeeze your pelvic and thigh muscles as often as you can remember. This again increases friction and pressure on his penis. Good for you. Good for him. Good result!**

your chances of having an orgasm during sex. So much so that the man who first brought the CAT to our attention in the early '90s, Edward Eichel, got a bit carried away and trumpeted it as the only guaranteed way to achieve simultaneous orgasm during sex.

Well, from experience and from anecdotal evidence I'd have to disagree. The CAT doesn't always deliver. According to Eichel's studies, however, 77 percent of females achieve orgasm "always or often" this way, and 36 percent of couples had simultaneous orgasms. Whatever, greater clitoral stimulation plus the judicial use of other techniques as needed has to mean that more women achieve more orgasms during intercourse. A good thing.

Ironically for the position that delivers the porn-star ideal—orgasm from penile penetration—the CAT is a wuss of a position. In a perverse way, I kind of like the idea that it's almost impossible to do while getting down and dirty.

What you can expect? Slow (very slow), gentle, and tender sex; a subtle dance between lovers.

What you can't expect? Absolutely no deep, hard, or fast thrusting or shouting of "Give it to me good, big boy." You'd actually feel a bit stupid shouting that during the CAT. It's more of an "I really love you"—"No, I really love you"—"Not as much as I love you" position. You get the picture.

If you and your lover are at the stage of intimacy (preliminary) where you can only have loud, dirty, and fast sex (oh, stop showing off) then the CAT is probably not worth bothering with. But if you're the sort of couple who cares enough to read this—in other words, you share a lot of intimacy and a lot of love, sometimes too much—then you'll be happy with the opportunity for lots of eye

Turn to IDEA 30, *Assume the position…*, for more on positions that improve stimulation for both partners.

Try another idea…

contact and prepared to give it the time it takes. You'll need it. Women: Don't even think of trying this if you're still angry with him for not doing the dishes.

SO GET ON BOARD

After assuming the missionary position, the man should move up the woman's body a few inches. His pelvis should be aligned with her vulva, directly over it. This means that only the tip of his penis is "in." This also means (and this is the whole point) that the greater part of his penis is pressing up against her vulva, pressing on her clitoris. Forget thrusting, think friction.

His legs should be together and straight; her legs should be wrapped around his thighs, with her ankles resting on his calves so her legs are as straight as possible. This means she will be opening her vagina and labia, again increasing friction. As a true gentleman, his weight would be taken on his elbows, but he may put his arms under her armpits and let himself rest gingerly on her.

"I blame my mother for my poor sex life. All she told me was, 'The man goes on top and the woman underneath.' For three years my husband and I slept on bunk beds."
JOAN RIVERS

Defining idea…

Now for the difficult part (you think I'm joking?): What you want to do is rock. No thrusting. She should tip her pelvis away from him down into the bed so his penis comes almost all the way out and then he should push down so he moves lower down her body and enters her fully. She tilts up to meet him, pulls her pelvis down so that he comes out again, and he pushes down with his pelvis so he moves back into her again. Her clitoris should be feeling constant pressure at all times. Carry on, and on, and on. Don't think of achieving orgasm, just get into the rhythmic dance. Don't thrust. Don't rush to orgasm. Slow and steady, that's the ticket. It's not easy, but when you get the rhythm it will all fall into place and feel natural. It helps if she sets the pace.

How was it for you?

Q   We tried the CAT. She came first. How can we guarantee simultaneous orgasm through intercourse alone?

A   *You can't. Nothing can. Keep practicing.*

Q   It felt good, but it took ages. Any refinements you could suggest?

A   *No time for the full-blown CAT? You can try what I call the "half-CAT." After assuming the missionary position she should close her legs so both feet are together with him still inside her. He should place his legs on either side of hers. This doesn't give the same clitoral stimulation as the CAT, but it does increase the pressure on the clitoris. The downside is that he'll fall out if he thrusts too hard. Another alternative is for the woman to get on top. She takes him inside her and then closes her legs as he opens his. Be careful now. She scoots up his body so she maximizes clitoral stimulation and then continues on as previously described.*

6

Make it a quick one

Do it right and a quickie can deliver the sort of thrills you haven't experienced since adolescence.

Many couples applaud the quickie—it fits nicely into their schedules. But it isn't really a "quickie" if it happens in bed. For the same amount of time or effort you could take your sex life to another level.

The essence of the quickie is surreptitiousness, not speed. The reason the quickie needs to be fast is not that you're supposed to be doing something else instead, like making Sunday dinner for the in-laws, but that at any moment your mother-in-law could pop her head around the kitchen door and offer to help with the gravy. Until you've had a quickie where there's every chance you could get caught in the flagrant act, you haven't really had a quickie at all.

Here's an idea for you... **Women: Initiating a quickie is a way to stay close to your partner during times when he's distant and you're busy. Women on the whole are pretty lousy at making men feel desired. We expect their never-ending sexual interest in us but don't reciprocate. There's nothing like initiating a quickie to make him feel desirable. It's the equivalent of him buying you a dozen roses.**

Doubt the aphrodisiac qualities of being caught? Think of all the couples you know who have maintained chronically dysfunctional but illicit "relationships" for years, convinced they're in the grip of a great passion. The truth is that they wouldn't have lasted five minutes if their sex life wasn't almost entirely sneaky and speedy. Quickies make for addictive sex.

Now, some people don't like quickies. They really don't. They might have gone along with it when you first got together because frankly they'd have had sex suspended from the Empire State Building if you seemed to think it was a good idea. But it's not really them and they don't feel comfortable if they think they'll get caught. They can't bear the thought of being embarrassed (usually men). They don't like getting messed up (usually women). And they don't even get an orgasm out of it (almost certainly women). So if your lover's in this category, you have to accept no gracefully or keep trying but be prepared for a lot of rejection. Alternatively, you could just get very good at persuading your partner that fast, hot sex up against a wall is the best idea they never had.

IMAGINE...

Any minute now you're expecting some guests to arrive. You're checking that the grill's hot enough or that you've got enough gin, when you catch sight of your partner passing by looking gorgeous. You reach for him, throw him against a wall, ravish him with kisses, hands roaming over and under clothes. Your lover is surprised, but begins to kiss you back passionately. You both go from zero to seventy in seconds. You glance at your watch. Your guests are expected to arrive in precisely five minutes. No time to undress. At any moment you could hear a ring on the doorbell. You fumble, push underwear aside, undo zips and buttons, reveal skin, pull clothes up and down so you achieve penetration. Fast and frantic sex is the only kind you've got time for. By the time your guests arrive, only a slight breathlessness gives away your secret.

Still not convinced? Read more about the aphrodisiac power of the element of surprise in IDEA 14, *Surprise!*

Try another idea...

ANY PROPS?

None. Except if you're a woman with a predilection for quickies it helps if you choose easily accessible underwear. There's something delicious about pushing aside the fabric and it adds to the erotic charge. Thongs are good, but the guy can end up with friction burns.

GOOD POSITION?

Standing up is the traditional "knee trembler," but this isn't terrific for any woman weighing more than a hundred pounds. It's even worse for her man. However, you don't have to go for the full monty. Instead of him taking the whole weight of your body, the woman can use a chair or table to support one leg. Or better still, he enters her from behind with her bent over slightly, so he has a good view of his penis entering. Grabbing her as she's going up the stairs and throwing her down on them gives you both some support, although it can be heavy on the rug burns.

"I love the lines men use. 'Please, I'll only put it in for a minute.' What am I? A microwave?"
BEVERLY MICKINS, comedian

Defining idea...

23

Q I'm not very comfortable with the idea of getting caught. It doesn't excite me; it makes me feel sick. Any suggestions?

A *Try the half-quickie. Its seductive power has nothing to do with getting caught but in making your partner feel that there's nothing in life you'd rather do than have sex with them. You just can't wait another minute! And that's a huge turn-on for anyone. The perfect scenario is when you're preparing to go out, ideally to a social event that's more important to you than your partner. Harass them about being punctual. Emphasize the importance of getting there with loads of time to spare. Get ready just a little bit earlier yourself so they feel slightly off-balance by your extreme punctuality. As you're hassling them out the front door, pause as if you've just remembered something and then, looking them straight in the eye, grab them and whisper, "Well, I guess they can wait another ten minutes." They should be delighted. If babysitters are involved then you'll have to be more adventurous. Garden shed? Car? Around the corner from the restaurant where you're meeting friends? Live a little. Just make sure you won't be surprised.*

Q I've initiated quickies twice and they've both been disasters. My partner was totally uninterested. What should I do next?

A *Ditch the getting caught element totally and instead concentrate on persuading your lover to have sex with you spontaneously in a place you wouldn't normally do it. If they don't go for that, he or she might just not like the whole idea. But you must discuss it. Why is your partner uninterested? Can he or she give good reasons that you understand? If you find it hard to discuss this, work on your communication with each other.*

7

Say it loud, say it proud— the art of talking dirty

I know. You can only bring yourself to talk dirty when you're drunk. Very drunk. So drunk that the next morning you can't remember what you said. That's why you need this idea.

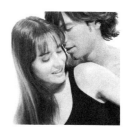

The right combination of pure filth whispered into your lover's ear at the right moment will catapult them into a thundering orgasm. But get it wrong, and they'll be running for the door.

Done right, a few lewd and lascivious words is the simplest way of making your sex life sing—no props or cost involved. If your sex style has been silent of late, don't suddenly unleash your potty-mouth persona without some warning, otherwise your partner will be perplexed at best, turned off at worst. As writer Brigid McConville points out in her book *Our Secret Lives*, there's a big taboo about talking about sex in our culture. Couples who start off filthy don't stay that way. She says, "The Big Ban on sex talk can start almost immediately in a relationship, intensifying to solid silence as the years go by. And by the time you've clocked up ten, twenty, or more years, it's a hard habit to break." So take it gently.

Here's an idea for you...

Talk dirty with conviction. Commit to your talk. Talking dirty comes easily when you're in the first few stages of lust, purely because talking dirty is easier with strangers. But when you've shared countless school meetings and fights over the remote, it's a lot harder. The other side of this is that you must try extra hard to support your lover's efforts. Don't undermine them with inopportune snickering.

FOUR WAYS TO ADD VALUE TO YOUR VERBAL

1. Give feedback

The most basic form of dirty talk is to describe what's happening to you and what it feels like. For example, "I love it when you kiss my collarbone like that." Or "It's such a turn-on watching your breasts from this angle." Giving a running commentary on what you're feeling and appreciating also serves to keep you "in the moment," making it less likely you'll start wondering who's going to get that promotion at work or if you have enough milk for breakfast. So encourage, praise, comment.

2. Build anticipation, make them beg

Tell your lover what you're going to do to them just before you do it. Ask them if they like it. Ask them if they don't. Ask them to ask nicely for what they want. Ask them to ask not so nicely. You get the idea. Before you know it, they're talking dirty, too. (However, use this tactic with discretion. Endless questioning can swiftly move from the sublime to the downright annoying, risking the passion-melting retort "Will you just get on with it?")

3. Role-play makes it easier—a lot easier—to talk dirty

Think how much easier it could be if you were pretending to be someone else . . .

4. Read bedtime stories to each other

It's not inhibition that gets in the way sometimes—it's lack of inspiration. After another hard day at the grind that's contemporary twenty-first-century life, making up a dirty scenario is just too much like hard work. That's when it pays to have a porn mag under the bed. Women are often turned on by stories geared toward men and soft porn will supply most couples with some inspiration for reading aloud.

But if that's too bold for you, there are erotic magazines and websites aimed at both sexes, such as Nerve.com. Or you could try reading a chapter a night from an erotica novel, which are aimed at exciting women but will also do the job for men. A classic for reading to each other is *My Secret Garden*, a collection of women's sexual fantasies by Nancy Friday.

For explosive orgasms, combine what you read here with IDEA 28, *Shortcuts to better orgasms*.

Try another idea...

FINAL WORD

Nobody can give you a script for talking dirty. Transcribed, it always sounds ridiculous. You need to develop your own style together. The main thing is to just do it. Once you start saying dirty words out loud—even if they're someone else's dirty words—you'll soon find your groove.

"If they call it 'dick,' don't call it 'hot, throbbing cock,' if they call it 'yoni,' don't call it 'gaping axe wound.' (In fact, don't ever call it that.) If in doubt use the basic anatomical name. You can get more creative later."
EM and LO, sex advice columnists on Nerve.com

Defining idea...

Q　**I can't build up the courage to talk dirty. I'd like to, but I doubt if my boyfriend would go for it, as he doesn't even talk. How can I do this without looking ridiculous?**

A　*The quiet lover isn't uncommon. If your partner is of the silent school of lovemaking then you may never get them to mutter filth in your ear. But you can try. First, concentrate on getting any noise out of them. Groan, moan, and whisper endearments while you come yourself and ask them to do the same for you. Tell them that a little non-verbal feedback will encourage your performance. After groans, work together on eliciting a few words. "Yes" and "please" are a start, and if you've been with a silent lover that will seem like a Shakespearean monologue!*

Q　**What if your partner talking dirty turns you off? Mine says things that make me feel a little sick, especially when he starts talking in a sort of baby talk and referring to my breasts as "titties."**

A　*It sounds as if he's either uncomfortable with talking dirty or thinks he's really good at it. If he's uncomfortable, you need to talk to him directly and find out if this is really turning him on or just his way of seeming willing. Tragically, it might be the second option: He thinks he's a wizard. Always be wary of those people who think they're really good at talking dirty. Inevitably, they're a little bit embarrassing, even if you love them. You need to retrain him, but you need to do it subtly. However, you shouldn't put up with that "titties" thing for a moment longer. We all have our personal pain threshold and he's stamping all over yours. Next time, look him in the eye, lower your voice an octave, and purr seductively, "Darling, I like to hear them called breasts." That should do it.*

8

Sleep is the new sex— honest!

I know a woman who tried to convince her lover that the really happening people were giving up sex in favor of sleep. But he wasn't buying it and neither am I!

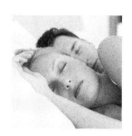

You'd like to have more sex, really you would. You're just too darn tired. Competitive tiredness between couples is a relatively new phenomenon and one result of both partners being strung out with exhaustion is no nookie.

Couples frazzled by the sheer weight of the goals they set themselves compete over how tired they are. You've worked for it and by god you've got it—a life so totally, overwhelmingly busy that you simply don't have the energy for sex.

It's not, of course, the end of a relationship if you go for some time with a lackluster or non-existent love life. Every relationship has its downtime. But the major worry with the tiredness excuse for avoiding sex is that it gains a weird sort of reverse momentum. Keep using tiredness as an excuse and before you know it, total inertia has set in. What you need is a two-pronged attack.

Here's an idea for you...

If sex usually takes place just before bed and is generally rushed and unsatisfying because you're both exhausted, make a weekly tryst for sex where you go to bed early and enjoy each other. Therapists agree that this "appointment system" is one of the easiest ways to ease you back into a good sex life.

FIRST PRONG—GET OVER YOURSELF

Here's a fact: Having sex when you're tired is not against the Geneva Convention. Having sex when you're tired can start off indifferently and get a whole lot better. And even if it doesn't, I'm firmly of the camp that believes that in a longstanding relationship, indifferent sex is better than no sex. At least you've got something to work on.

If you're of the aficionado brigade who would rather not bother unless sex is a multiorgasmic garden of delight, then you have to negotiate this with your partner. Make definite dates when you're going to do it. Make sex that day your priority. See it as a red-letter event.

SECOND PRONG—REORGANIZE YOUR WORKLOAD

This is anecdotal, based purely on my experience of knowing a lot of couples in their thirties with young children and having no sex. At the root of it is usually resentment on the part of one partner toward the other. Generally the woman is resentful of the man. She is often working, even if only part-time, and doing most of the childcare, too. Women who have given up work to look after their children tend not to be as resentful, but they feel that their men don't appreciate all that they do. This is my experience but it's backed up by at least two recent surveys.

Defining idea...

"He said, 'I can't remember when we last had sex.' And I said, 'Well, I can and that's why we ain't doing it.'"
ROSEANNE BARR

WHO DOES THE MOST AFTER A HARD DAY'S WORK?

Read IDEA 44, *It's not all in your mind*—there may be medical reasons for your tiredness.

Try another idea...

This quiz gives couples a quick visual reference of who does more around the home. Mark the gender of the partner who most often undertakes a particular task. This test can be an eye-opener for couples that think they have a pretty equal relationship. If it's not so equal, you have to take steps to delegate or equalize your workload, or your sex life is unlikely to get back to normal any time soon.

	M	F
Getting the children ready for the day	☐	☐
Making breakfast	☐	☐
Making packed lunches	☐	☐
Taking children to school or bus stop	☐	☐
Supervising homework	☐	☐
Teacher's meetings	☐	☐
Immunizations, trips to the doctor	☐	☐
Dealing with childcare	☐	☐
Bathing children and getting them ready for bed	☐	☐
Bedtime stories	☐	☐
Arranging play dates with other parents	☐	☐
Grocery shopping	☐	☐
Cooking evening dinner	☐	☐
Cleaning up at the end of the evening	☐	☐
Paying bills	☐	☐
Home repairs	☐	☐
Cleaning	☐	☐
Taking out garbage	☐	☐

Buying children's clothes	M ☐	F ☐
Washing and drying clothes	M ☐	F ☐
Loading the dishwasher	M ☐	F ☐
Gardening	M ☐	F ☐
Maintaining and cleaning car	M ☐	F ☐
Organizing social life	M ☐	F ☐

You might be reading this and thinking, "I'm the major breadwinner. I work my butt off and can't do childcare, too." But you'll have to find some compromise for the sake of your relationship. You need to talk openly about how you divide your joint workload, give each other the space to have a life as an individual, and find time to spend as a couple. If you're reading this and thinking, "Who needs a quiz to tell me I do it all?" then stop and examine your martyr-syndrome. Yes, you've got one. At all costs, you have to get rid of it or "I'm just so tired" will sound the death knell for your sex life.

Overprotective parents take note: Someone else can very well look after your children. Your relationship with each other can't be tended by anyone else but the two of you.

Workaholics take note: Quit your job tomorrow and someone else will fill your job/role/career by Monday morning. No one else can take your place in your relationship.

Q **Your advice to make a date for sex just felt like another thing to add to my to-do list. Isn't this approach a bit, well, functional?**

How was it for you?

A *Yes, I can see why you'd think that. And it's not that I'm unsympathetic, but my point is that you can't rely on spontaneity and lust to propel you into sex. My advice to you is the same as to women who are pregnant and aren't interested in sex. Indeed, it's the only advice I give to pregnant women (who ask!): Stop relying on your hormones, start relying on your man. Relaxing and giving your partner the chance to get you in the mood can often work wonders. Promise yourself that you'll let him do his darnedest to haul you from lethargy and you'll be amazed how often it actually works and you feel your libido stirring. If, after ten minutes or so of foreplay, he still can't persuade you that sex is more worthwhile than sleep, too bad, you'll just have to break it to him gently that tonight he's flying solo. Nine times out of ten, however, you'll have sex.*

Q **We have small kids and both work full-time. We barely see each other, much less make love. Any fire-lighting tips?**

A *The best piece of advice I ever received on keeping the home fires burning was from a sophisticated woman in her forties. She had a grown-up family and a gorgeous husband who was devoted to her after twenty-five years of marriage despite (to my certain knowledge) a host of young women's desperate attempts to seduce him. When I asked her how they kept interest in each other after so long she told me, "Well, darling, we always make a point of going to bed at the same time as each other—early, around ten. [Significant pause] And I always get into bed naked." Try it.*

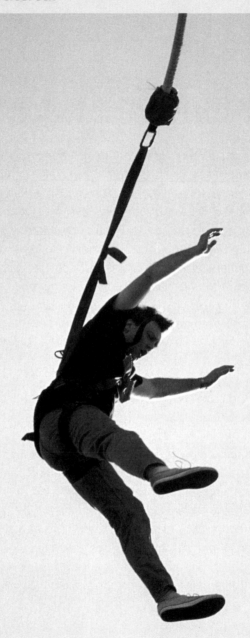

Get over yourself

If bungee jumping could do for us what sex can, we'd be lining up to try it.

There are minor and major reasons for periods when we don't want sex much. Sometimes we simply can't be bothered.

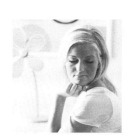

Answer yes or no to these questions:

1. Do you enjoy sex when you get going and then think, "We should do this more often"?
2. Are there any physical reasons you avoid sex?
3. Are there any psychological reasons you avoid sex?
4. Do you simply prefer to read gardening catalogs or watch *American Idol* than have sex?

If you answered yes to questions 2 and 3, then this idea isn't going to help. If you answered yes to 1 and 4 then it's time for some tough love. You owe it to your body to have sex, you owe it to your psyche to have sex, and you almost certainly owe it to your relationship.

In a long-term relationship, wanting sex is a mind thing as much as a physical imperative. The next time you sense a resistance to the idea of sex, remember the

Here's an idea for you...

If you're feeling down, try having sex. Sex releases hormones that have an antidepressant effect so it could prove a real comfort to you when you're blue. It's an especially powerful way to express painful emotions, and couples sometimes find that it helps them recover from traumatic experiences such as bereavement.

words of Tom Hopkins, bestselling author of *How to Master the Art of Selling*: "Winners almost always do what they think is the most productive thing possible at every given moment: losers never do." Sometimes, he says, the most productive use of your time is to watch the sunset or talk to your spouse. Usually, I say, the most productive use of your time is having sex. Done well, with passion and enthusiasm, half an hour of sex is worth hours of doing just about anything else—it's the ultimate multitasking activity. It's not just good for your relationship; it's great for you, too. When you're dithering about whether or not to go for it, reread this chapter and remember all that sex can do for you. Then ask, "Am I a winner or a loser?"

Your mission
To overcome a "take it or leave it" attitude to sex.

Your task
Read the following every day for the next week and thereafter once a week.

SEX DEFUSES STRESS

"Progressive relaxation" is a relaxation technique that involves tensing and then relaxing muscles in a controlled manner throughout the body. After a while, it sends you to sleep. Orgasmic sex works in much the same way. (No snarky comments, please.) It also involves tensing and relaxing your muscles, but far more intensely. The result is that people with fulfilling sex lives are generally far less stressed, less anxious, less hostile, and, bizarrely, far more likely to take responsibility for their own lives (one of the prime signs of a successful person, apparently).

Read IDEA 44, *It's not all in your mind*, if you're bemused by where your libido's gone.

Try another idea...

SEX BOOSTS SELF-ESTEEM

Good sex makes us feel better about ourselves because it can be such an intimate experience. You're letting your soul out for a little play in front of another person, and it's a huge ego kick if they like what they see. It gives our personality a sense of completeness that we rarely experience unless we're particularly evolved human beings. Of course, if you don't receive wholehearted acceptance, the opposite happens and you feel

"Sex is not the answer. Sex is the question. Yes is the answer."
ANONYMOUS

Defining idea...

lousy. This is why you shouldn't have sex with people who don't seem to like you letting your soul out to play or, even worse, are so self-absorbed they don't seem to notice that's what you're doing. But, hey, that's a whole different book.

SEX IS THERAPEUTIC

The Chinese believe that you can treat everything from a cold to eczema with sex. One thing for sure, it's good for your heart both metaphorically and literally. One study looked at the sex lives of women who had been admitted to the hospital following a heart attack. Of these, 65 percent reported that they experienced no sexual feelings or were unhappy with their sex lives in some way. When researchers asked women who were hospitalized for other, non–heart-related conditions, only 24 percent reported having nonexistent or poor-quality sex lives.

37

SEX IS CREATIVE

In an ideal world we'd all be scribbling away in diaries or expressing our emotions through dance and no doubt we'd be a happier, less repressed society for it. But who would feed the cat?

Seriously though, most of us don't make time to express our emotions or even to recognize them as they flit across our consciousness. During sex is a perfect time to get back in touch with the "inner you." As you touch each other, imagine you're expressing how you feel right at that moment. How are you feeling? Angry, sad, happy, secure, frustrated? Communicate this to your lover through your touch, words, and actions. For some, this will appear scarier than the thought of dressing up in a diaper and parading down Main Street, and you're the ones who really need to experiment with sex as a creative act.

SEX HELPS YOU LIVE LONGER

It's true. Studies have shown that those with a healthy sex life are more resistant to disease and the ill effects of stress. An orgasm boosts the body's white cell count (the cells that fight infection) by up to 20 percent. But note that we're talking about a happy sex life here. Miserable, joyless sex probably doesn't confer benefits, although no one has done the studies. We don't know why good sex works, but it's probably partly to do with the beneficial effects of having someone stroke you lovingly. Your immune system improves when you're caressed, stroked, and hugged.

Q   **Are you saying we should grit our teeth, think of the advantages, and have sex when we don't feel like it?**

How was it for you?

A   *Exactly. "Feeling" like sex is a fragile flower that rarely blooms. Forget feeling like it, just do it. There are all sorts of complex psychological reasons why we stop having sex with our long-term partners. Allow this to happen and inertia will set in. This idea is aimed at reversing that mind-set, which is why you have to read about the benefits of sex repeatedly. It's a brainwashing thing.*

Q   **My partner and I are perfectly happy with doing it once a month or so. Are we damaging our health?**

A   *If you and your partner are both totally happy with little or no sex, fine. But if there's any sort of discrepancy (and I guess you wouldn't be reading this if you were both happy), then work a little harder at getting yourself in the mood more often. Think more about sex, do more to pleasure yourself, make your daily life as sensual as possible. If the problem is that your partner doesn't deliver what you need to enjoy sex, then you have to talk to him or her, but above all remember that sex is one of those things where "use it or lose it" applies in spades.*

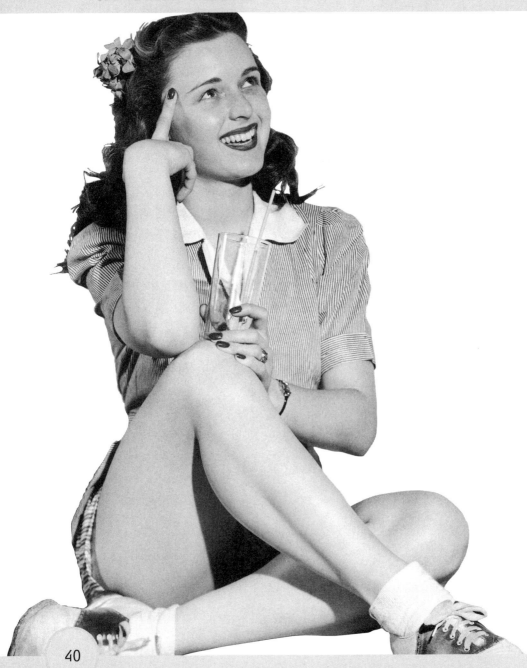

10

Get jiggy with your G-spot

Think of the G-spot like Wilmer Valderrama's sex appeal. It might not do much for you, but that doesn't mean it doesn't exist.

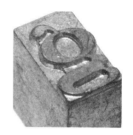

It's generally accepted that it was Freud and the '50s who did it for the G-spot.

Stimulation of this internal hot spot, situated just inside the vagina, can result in the so-called vaginal orgasm. But when Freud branded clitoral orgasms "immature" and vaginal orgasms as superior he guaranteed that come the sexual revolution a whole swathe of stubborn women, relieved that they could come at all, weren't going to waste a precious moment fixating on an elusive vaginal orgasm and dissing their lovely clitoral ones because some dead guy thought they weren't good enough.

The clitoral orgasm got to be the popular girl at the party while the vaginal orgasm languished in a corner. Even the sexologists gave up on her. Here's one example: "It is clear that women only have one kind of climax—even though different climaxes brought about in different ways can feel different. And...this climax is brought about by one thing only—the arousal of the clitoris."

Here's an idea for you... **If you want to be able to ignore the sensation of needing to pee while searching for your G-spot, empty your bladder beforehand and anything that comes out will be ejaculate.**

So, even if you were one of the 30 percent of women who claimed to come through penetration, the general opinion was that you were either misguided or showing off. Then came the '90s and it became fashionable to "give bi a try" and a whole generation of young women went home from their girlfriends to teach their boyfriends what they'd learned. However, a lot of older, more sexually experienced women—through trial and error with their long-term male lovers—discovered that the G-spot was alive and kicking, but weren't making a fuss about it.

OK, sociology lesson over, but it's fascinating to think there are fashions in orgasm just like everything else. Anyway, here's what we think now. Most (if not all) women have a G-spot. Some people experience terrific sexual excitement from having their G-spot stimulated. Some feel a warm oozy feeling like listening to carols at Christmas—and just about as sexually exciting. Some find G-spot stimulation intensely irritating. Some feel nothing much at all. And some feel an overwhelming need to pee that, depending on their sexual makeup, feels either unbearably uncomfortable or unbearably exciting. The only way you're going to find out if your G-spot is worth bothering with is to try it out.

There's good and bad news for guys who are reading this and getting excited at the thought of a female orgasm initiated by penetrative sex. The good news? This really is a case of size doesn't matter—the G-spot is situated within the first three inches of the vagina. The bad news? Humping away is going to miss the spot entirely. Your lady won't come from deep, hard thrusting in the time-honored tradition of porn movies. It requires shallow penetration, skill, and a bit of a concentration to hit the G-spot with your penis, much less get her off in this way.

For more ways to make the G-spot happy turn to IDEA 36, *The joy of shopping*, and IDEA 37, *Play away.*

Try another idea...

WOMEN...

Squat and feel it out. The G-spot is situated on the front of the vaginal wall about a third to halfway toward the cervix, a few inches inside. It feels slightly rough and is about a couple of centimeters across. Struggling? Feel for something that's more of a ridge than round. Pressing on the G-spot will feel spongy because what you're feeling through the skin of the vaginal wall is the insulation that surrounds the urethra, which carries urine from your bladder to the outside world. The insulating sheath includes multiple glands that swell during sexual excitement and when stimulated in the right way will spurt out a clear fluid that emerges through the urethra just like pee. This is totally different in composition from pee and is, in fact, the so-called female ejaculate.

Many people don't like the idea of women ejaculating. And many of these people are women. But sisters, relax. Embrace your bodily fluids. Even if you don't want to go the whole way, playing around with our G-spot is a pleasurable thing for most. Many people can get a big hit from just fiddling around down there. Many aren't men.

"Sex pleasure in the woman is a kind of magic spell; it demands complete abandon; if words or movements oppose the magic of caresses the spell is broken."
MASTERTON and COLDWELL, *How to Drive Your Man Wild in Bed*

Defining idea...

MEN…

Men who want to float their partner's love boat with some G-spot action might find using a finger rather than their penis is a lot less tiring. Have your partner sit or lie facing you, insert your index finger, and press firmly repeatedly. You may have to go quite fast, but if she likes this, get her to demonstrate first or you could do her damage. Also, try hooking your finger slightly as if beckoning and press repeatedly on the G-spot.

If you get bored and decide to employ your love wand in your quest, remember that shallow penetration is the only kind that works and imagine you're aiming for the navel. Rear entry positions are best; the "spoon," where you both lie on your sides with him behind her, is easiest on both of you. Nothing happening? Try a vibrator that's specifically designed to hit the G-spot. Women may feel the need to pee during these maneuvers, as stimulating the G-spot means you're pressing on the urethra. But stick with it, as it means you're getting close.

Is it worth it? Nearly all women enjoy having attention paid to the anterior wall of the vagina because of the huge number of nerve endings there. Becoming aware of how they react to different kinds of stimulation—manual, penile, and plastic—can only improve your sexual repertoire of sensations. Just don't get hung up on it. Women don't need another body part to get neurotic about.

Q   **We kept at it for ten minutes. Nothing much happened though I enjoyed it. Was that long enough?**

A   *Plenty long enough for the first attempt. Try again when you're having a particularly long and animalistic session and you're very steamed up. The more excited you are the better. Performance pressure won't help, so buy a vibrator and experiment on your own.*

Q   **We couldn't find it. What are we doing wrong?**

A   *When you're searching for the G-spot together, plenty of foreplay is crucial. It swells when its owner is sexually excited and you can't find it otherwise. So, when she's well on the way to coming, apply firm, steady pressure to the G-spot. There's actually another hot spot just above the G-spot between it and the cervix. Try experimenting with the anterior wall of the vagina in general. You might be surprised at what you discover.*

How was it for you?

45

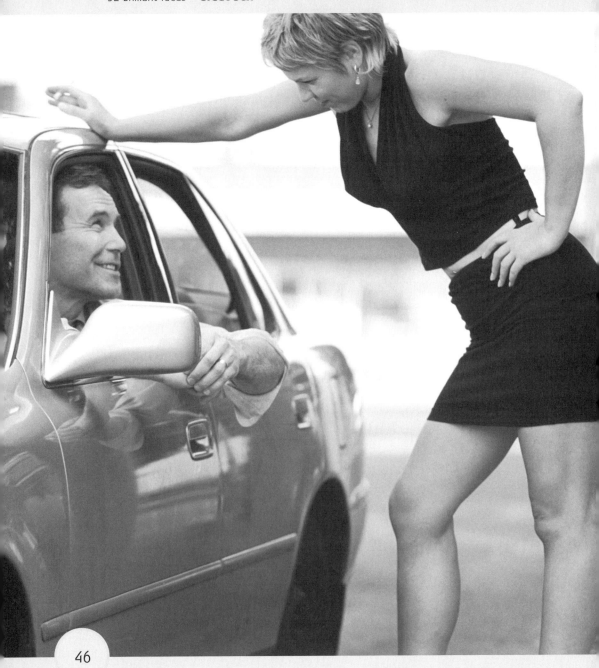

11

Paying for it

Slutty sex can be a turn-on for both of you.

Both sexes can get a huge kick out of acting out prostitution fantasies. This explores our attitudes toward power and control (often erotically charged) and both sexes are able to relish the freedom of imagining that they're having no-holds-barred, no-strings-attached sex.

The "client" gets the thrill of the clean transaction, of the freedom of asking for what he wants, of control, of being in charge. The "whore" gets the visible proof that he values what she does in bed. (For the sake of clarity, I'm being traditional and assuming he is the client and she is the whore but, of course, this fantasy begs for role reversal. The powerful female client and the stud-for-hire can be just as much of a turn-on.)

This is one that definitely works better if you've both had a couple of drinks beforehand because alcohol removes the self-consciousness from role-playing, and for this idea to really work you both need to stay in character throughout.

Here's an
idea for
you...

There's an easy way to add a heightened sense of reality to the fantasy of paid-for sex: She keeps the money.

ACTING OUT

1. The Classic

Arrange to meet on a certain street corner at a certain time. Make sure there's not the slightest chance of it being mistaken for a red-light area or you might get more reality than you bargained for. She should dress as overtly sexy as she feels comfortable with in public; simply slipping off her panties beforehand will give that added frisson. At the appointed hour, he pulls up in his car and asks whether she is available. She replies, "For what?" Then he tells her in explicit detail. She comes back with the cost. Haggling or "negotiating a price" can be a turn-on, and she shouldn't get in the car until the deal is done. You can now either drive back home and pretend it's her place or, if you're daring, use the car (somewhere private, of course, or again this game could get a bit too real).

2. The Pick-up

She's sitting at a hotel bar, looking sexy but demure. It helps if she adopts a slightly different look from usual—more makeup, hair slightly different, heels higher—a look that makes her feel unlike herself. She should make sure her underwear is brand new—nothing he's ever seen before. She should order a different drink from usual and adopt a different name and personality—the easier the new persona comes to her the more convincing this will be. The same applies to him: He should invent a new persona, too, and "work it up."

He approaches her and, although there may be some preliminary small talk, eventually a conversation not unlike the one above has to take place. Maintain eye contact. It's sexier. When you're done head home (or better still, take a room). Don't talk too much.

3. The Hotel Room

Book a hotel room and pay for it in advance.

She arrives first and changes—a wig if she can bear it, lingerie he's never seen before, heels, different perfume, negligée if she's uncomfortable strutting around nearly naked. Make the mood seductive with music and candles. She should psyche herself up—she's a high-class call girl and her job is to make him feel good. High-class call girls are paid a lot because they're great actresses, so she should put her heart into it.

At last, he knocks on the door and she lets him in. Introduce yourselves by different names. Open a bottle of champagne. He can be nervous—that's still in character. But she must be confident and tease, flirt, or be sexually voracious. She should read her client and take her clues from him (he, of course, has to act out his other side— the side that frequents prostitutes). She must make it clear she's here for one reason only—to give him the best sexual experience he's ever had. What would it take? What does he like? She should name her price and make it high. She's the ultimate indulgence. She's *expensive*. When the price has been agreed on and she has the cash, she should lead him to the bed and get down to business. She should remember that this is her job and she's very, very good at it. If she can slip a few tricks in that he definitely won't be expecting, all the better. Maintain roles until the door closes behind him.

Combine this with what you read in IDEA 15, *Something for the weekend*. Going away can be the perfect scenario for putting this idea into action.

Try another idea...

"You always pay for sex, but not always in cash."
ANONYMOUS

Defining idea...

49

How was
it for
you?

Q I think the paid-for-sex fantasy is distasteful. Am I being unduly prudish?

A *Women who charge for sex exert a powerful fascination for many people—but maybe not for you. However, I know from interviewing men talking about their sexual fantasies that the idea of being with a prostitute makes completely faithful men wonder, "What if?" And women—even the most feminist—get an illicit thrill at the thought of breaking one of our society's strongest taboos and making themselves completely sexually available. Since in our culture women decide whom they'll sleep with and when, there's something powerfully erotic in subverting that societal law by pretending she has no choice but to offer herself as a sexual plaything to anyone who can afford her. The pretended helplessness is a huge turn-on for many women, whether you approve or not. Turn the page if there's an issue in your past that makes thinking about prostitution unpleasant or even painful, and I'm sorry it's offended you. But if not, dip a toe in. What offends us pushes our boundaries, and that is powerfully erotic.*

Q We enjoyed the sex, but the lead up was awkward. Any ideas?

A *Try again. Introduce some new elements to the initial pick-up or try reversing roles. Promise to do all you can to support each other in the make-believe. No giggling or snickering. Also, next time promise each other you'll each do one thing that the other one isn't expecting during the encounter. After all, you're supposed to be strangers and you'd surprise each other in real life. If none of these suggestions work, then maybe this just isn't your scenario. Move on.*

12

The love's there, but the lust's gone AWOL

Hey, sexual pioneer! Yes, we're talking to you.

If you're a baby boomer in a sexual relationship that's lasted more than nine years, then you're breaking new sexual ground. The human race doesn't have much practice doing what you're doing. We simply don't know how to do long-term relationships.

As Dr. Alan Altman writes in *Making Love the Way We Used To, Or Better*, "Many people are disappointed when they can't re-create those early thrilling feelings. We don't really have many examples of how to keep a twenty-five-plus year marriage alive sexually. At the turn of the century a forty-seven-year-old male was considered old."

Are we programmed to get bored with a long-term partner? There's a persuasive argument that we are. Psychologists believe that one reason we lose interest in sex with long-term lovers is the powerful anti-incest taboos that are part of nearly every culture. Basically, in a "functional" family, brothers and sisters who are brought up

Here's an idea for you...

A long-term sexual relationship will go in cycles—sometimes strong, sometimes fading. Sexual desire is something you can rekindle, but make sure your partner is singing from the same hymn sheet. When the first flush of lust passes, it won't come back without will and compassion from each of you for the other.

together aren't attracted to each other despite incredible proximity. However, brothers and sisters who are brought up apart often are. It may be that if we live too long with someone of the opposite sex, we stop reacting to their sexual charisma. This is why we must never get too cozy with each other or allow our boundaries to become too melded.

We long for the thrills of the beginning of the relationship. We yearn for the time when our partners were crazy for us. Sometimes we want it so much that we move onto another relationship to get the kicks. So there's the bad news. Your challenge is to decide what to do about it. Interview the sexual pioneers—women and men who have successfully lived with each other for many years—and they talk touchingly about the power that sexuality shared with one partner over many years can hold. One woman interviewed by writer Brigid McConville in her book *The Secret Life* says, "We have been together for so long, when I look at him not just as my aging bloke but as the man who made love to me on the beach in Greece, on the train across Europe, and tied to the bedposts in a hotel in Spain. No one else has those intimate memories, just us. No one else knows what he is capable of. It's a bond so strong it's a bit like having children together: Nothing can change the history of our intimacy and what we have made and shared and I can conjure up images of us making love together any time I like."

How do you get to the place where a lifetime's worth of loving experience informs your view of your lover? In a nutshell, don't get boring and don't get bored. Ask yourself some hard questions. If you love your partner but are no longer excited by them, reverse it. How exciting are you? How passionate are you? Would you be attracted to yourself? Do you feel alive?

For more on remaining your own person and keeping a spark between you turn to IDEA 39, *Let a woman be a woman and a man be a man*, and IDEA 47, *Developing sexual mystique*.

Try another idea...

Are you passionate about work or your interests? Do you have any interests? Are you enthusiastic about your children, your friends, and the things you talk about with them?

What projects do you have on the back burner for the future that excite you?

If you're drawing a blank here, it's time to get back your passion for life. There's absolutely no way you'll get it back for your partner without it. And be warned, moving onto another partner in the hope of regaining your passion for life will work in the short term, but never in the long term. This isn't always the complete answer to the "love but no lust" dilemma, but it's the first crucial step.

"Anyone who knows Dan Quayle knows that he would rather play golf than have sex any day."
MARILYN QUAYLE, responding to charges that her husband had an affair while on a golf trip

Defining idea...

How was it for you?

Q How do you rekindle your passion for life when you have no time?

A *If you don't make time for this it means it's not your priority, which is a little sad. One simple way that was taught to me by a very wise woman with five kids and a work schedule to make you cry is to put down all tools—whether computer, iron, or dishwasher—at 8:30 p.m. each night. That means the house is often a mess and I sometimes have to rise early, sit in the car to get away from the children, and finish work I should have done the night before. But, and it's a big but, I get time nearly every night to chill out on my own (usually), with my partner (often), or with friends (occasionally). Yes, even on a weeknight. Just find an hour a day at first to get back your juice and take it from there. At first, you'll be twiddling your thumbs and thinking, "I really should clean the bathroom." However, soon you'll be yearning for your hour like water in the desert.*

Q Our sex is fine, but it's just not earth-shattering. Why not?

A *It won't always be, but you can feel as sexually alive as you did at the beginning of the relationship, even more so. The secret is not to rely on spontaneous desire. If you want exciting sex, you have to become an expert at making it happen. The reasons we lose interest when it's proscribed by society and not "forbidden," i.e., when we're "settled down," are huge and complex—we've just touched on them here. Fight your conditioning. There are plenty of ways to combat sexual inertia, but the best advice is to stop waiting for fireworks to just happen. Think about sex, reach for sex, want sex, relish sex. Use it to give life texture and make it fun.*

13

Touchy-feely

Learn to express sensuality with your whole body.

Think of ways you can actively be more aware of your bodies and new sensations together. Here are some ideas to keep you both sensually oriented throughout the next week.

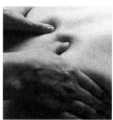

STEP 1

Showering together is one of those things you do at the beginning of a relationship that tails off as the mortgage gets bigger and your hair gets grayer. Give your lover a surprise this week. Wait until it's good and steamy in there. Strip off, step in, and start soaping them down.

I recommend showers rather than baths. Although I'm seriously addicted to candlelit baths, when you're getting wet together I think there's something more intimate about showering than bathing. Probably because the sound of the shower cuts you off from the outside world, makes talk less likely, and forces you to get physical together. But only, of course, if your shower is a powerful one. A pathetic dribble where you are both edging the other one out to get a share of the water is a

Here's an idea for you... **Men: Instead of using your hands to massage her body, use the sensitive inside of your forearms—it will feel new for both of you.**

waste. If you're looking for a good reason to install a decent shower, make it your love life.

Note for women: Put on some gorgeous wispy underwear and step into the shower with him when he's not expecting it. Naked's good. Naked's great. But the feel (and the look!) of the wet fabric plastered against your slick body and the rush he'll get from pushing it aside to get at you should make for a different kind of experience.

STEP 2

Look for different ways to surprise each other with unexpected sensations.

- Wear something different from the norm. If you sleep naked, try silk pajama bottoms. If you always wear a nightdress, change to a simple white cotton panty and tank top.

- Introduce a feather into lovemaking. Ask your lover to close his eyes and trail it over his bare skin. Some people hate it, some love it, but it sensitizes bare skin and makes it more reactive to other stimulation.

- Heat up a towel with a hair dryer while your lover's bathing and offer it to her as she comes out. A toasty hot towel is delicious, unexpected, and will get you Brownie points for thoughtfulness. Make sure she does the same for you.

- While you're making love, rub an ice cube over your lover's bare back or nipples until it melts. Take in the sensations, from shock through enjoyment. Add some gentle slaps if you want to get kinky. Heat, then cold, is very sensitizing.

STEP 3

Turn to IDEA 34, *The love bath*, for some more things to do in the shower. IDEA 45, *Pressure– it's not a dirty word*, gives details of massage techniques.

Try another idea...

Marilyn Monroe's sexual signature note had nothing to do with her looks (her partner couldn't see her) or his degree of sexual satisfaction (he didn't even come) and everything to do with the electrifying power that touch can have on your average adult male, deprived as he is of all-over, deeply sensual, touch.

Marilyn, so the story goes, would ask her lover to lie on his front and remain very, very still. Once he was in position she'd straddle him from behind and whisper in his ear that he was going to help her to come. Then she'd liberally apply oil on his back and her body and start slithering up and down on him, rubbing her vulva and clitoris against his back and buttocks, over and over again, finding just the right spot to grind her hips to give her the right pressure, whispering all the time about how turned on she was, how hot she was, how close she was...until, finally, inevitably, she came. The guy probably quite enjoyed it, too.

Clever Marilyn—what's more likely to make your lover mad for you than letting them know they're driving you mad with lust, while ensuring they get to have a nice little rest at the same time?

"I'm suggesting we call sex something else, and it should include everything from kissing to sitting close together."
SHERE HITE, sex researcher

Defining idea...

57

Women: Try your own version of the Marilyn maneuver.

Men: To reawaken your sense of touch (the point of this exercise), you could massage your lover while asking her to stay perfectly still. Once she's melting, use your imagination, and her body, to find a way of bringing yourself to the point of orgasm without her having to lift a finger. Extra points if you manage to come, but if you don't, make sure she does.

How was it for you?

Q   My partner finds this sort of stuff excruciating. He even finds taking a shower together a bit irritating rather than interesting. What can I do?

A   *He's a man deeply in denial of something, although I have no idea what. Some of the scenarios in this book can make men feel very self-conscious and foolish. It's a difficult one. What he has to understand is that it's not about him—it's about you. Is he prepared to give a little to make you happy? That should be reason enough for him to try it. Be patient and in the meantime treat yourself sensually every chance you get. Ask him to share in that with you. Eventually you'll break him down.*

Q   This is all very nice but does it really help improve our sex life?

A   *You're right. Waving a feather over your skin isn't going to produce any thundering orgasms. But becoming more aware of the power of touch will make you more sensitive during lovemaking and more likely to experiment. Following these ideas or similar ones will open up communication between you. You'll be a better lover. And that's guaranteed to improve your sex life.*

14

Surprise!

Isn't it time you got in touch with your creative side?

Laura Corn, author of *101 Nights of Grrreat Sex*, has based her considerable bestselling success on one simple concept: the importance of the surprise factor. Each of her 101 suggestions depends on the fact that your partner doesn't have a clue what sexual delight you're planning.

It's a clever gimmick and it works. Surprise your lover sexually every week for a year and you can bet your booty you won't be collecting any "boring in bed" prizes. Encouraging the element of surprise in your sex life will keep you young and playful, keep you feeling cherished and appreciated, and keep your lover crazy for you.

Here's an idea for you...

Do something slightly different *every* time you make love. Throw in an element of surprise. Mixing it up will become second nature after a few weeks and the payoff will make it worthwhile.

A little bit of effort to surprise your lover with a new technique, seduction, outfit, or behavior reaps huge improvements. As long as it's something unexpected, the surprise can be whatever you like. It can be filthy, funny, sweet, and romantic, or it can be more embarrassing than karaoke night.

WHY SURPRISE WORKS

Some of your surprises will be easy to organize. Some will take more planning. You might spend an hour (or more) setting up a gorgeous seduction for your mate, which is a lot I grant you, but the end result (and this is no exaggeration) will be burned into the hard drive of their memory for the rest of their life. Great sex has that sort of effect on us.

But even more unforgettable for your mate than the great sex you'll enjoy is how loved they'll feel. Men, just as much as women (in fact, if the psychologists are to be believed, even *more* than women), are delighted by the proof that someone wants them so much that they'll put thought and effort into their seduction. All of us love to feel special.

WHAT DOES IT TAKE FOR IT TO WORK?

It takes both of you to commit to the idea. You will only want to put effort into thrilling your partner if you feel they're going to make the same effort for you.

It will be especially hard to have a boring sex life if you combine this idea with IDEA 17, *Learn the art of kaizen.*

Try another idea...

I recommend Laura Corn's book (previously mentioned) because she gives you lots of ideas and she gives you structure. The surprise element can't be spontaneous, at least not at first. If we don't plan, we just get lazy and don't bother. You're aiming to give your lover a "guaranteed surprise," if you see what I mean. In other words, although they'll be able to look forward to being surprised, they won't know what they're looking forward to.

If you don't want to spring for Corn's book, then in the immortal words of Fleetwood Mac, "Go your own way." Or simply customize some of the following suggestions to get the ball rolling:

"We want to know how to turn our mates on. We want them to know what turns us on. We'd like more variety...more foreplay...more surprises...more interest...new tricks...and, once in a while, somebody else should do all the work!"
LAURA CORN

Defining idea...

61

For her

■ He's in the shower. Wait until it's good and steamy in there and then slip in beside him wearing your flimsiest, sheerest underwear. If there's one thing more likely to turn him on than you naked, it's wet, clinging wisps of material. (Guys could try this, too, but it has to be silk boxers—soggy, cotton tighty-whiteys just don't cut it.)

■ On your next date, you can keep your coat on. Well, you don't want the whole restaurant to know you're naked underneath. Just him.

For him

■ Buy her half a case of her favorite wine (a dozen bottles is classier, but might be too much of a demand on your imagination). Around the neck of each, place a sealed envelope containing details of where and when you're going to drink it together. These are IOUs of pleasure. Let your imagination run riot.

■ One night when you're getting amorous in a lovey-dovey sort of way, suddenly flip personality—change the whole atmosphere, from Dr. Jekyll to Mr. Hyde. Stop smiling. Get mean. Overcome her. Tie her wrists to the headboard and blindfold her. Now you can do whatever you like, but if you want to give her a night to remember (and especially if she's still really pissed off with you), go down on her until she stops cursing and starts begging.

■ Spend an hour or so pleasuring her sensually, such as oral sex, washing her hair, painting her toenails, applying body lotion to every inch of her skin, or holding her and stroking her hair until she falls asleep. Don't allow her to do a thing for you in return.

Q **I tried getting a little rough, but my wife hated it. How should I approach this now?**

How was it for you?

A *The all-important point of this whole surprise thing is that it shouldn't come as a surprise to your mate. You need to talk beforehand and agree on the general concept of bringing the element of surprise into your lovemaking. If it came out of the blue, being tied up could easily be too much. Surprise her with a few less extreme ideas, then talk to her about her feelings on bondage to establish whether the bondage per se was the problem or whether it was your personality change that shocked her.*

Q **I bought my wife some expensive lingerie and laid it out on the bed. She laughed and said she'd save it for "a big occasion." What did I do wrong?**

A *She probably felt pressured. Be careful not to make the surprise simply about the lingerie. Make it about* her *in the lingerie. In fact, forget about the lingerie for a while and concentrate on giving her a massage next time she's tired. Surprise her with romance and thoughtfulness for a few weeks, then explain how you're trying to improve your relationship. If she seems uncomfortable, suggest that maybe she could surprise you with the lingerie sometime, if she feels like it. Remember, no pressure. Hand the reins to her then continue with the romance, the thoughtfulness, and the occasional move in bed that she's not expecting. Soon she'll be joining in.*

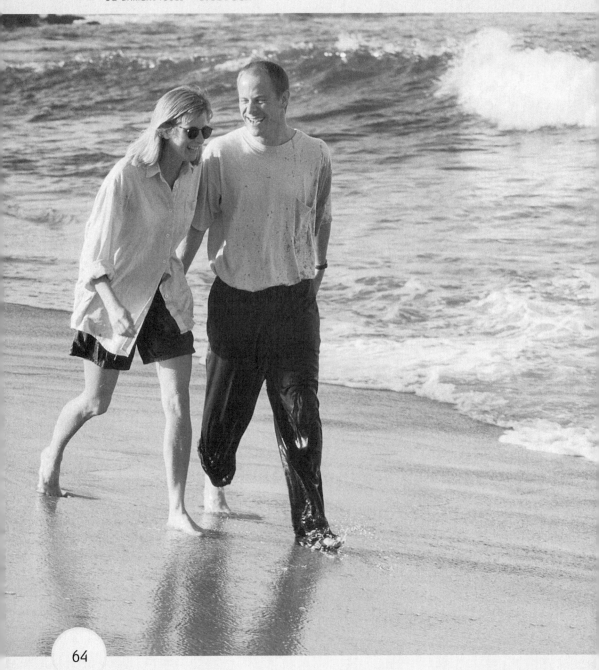

15

Something for the weekend

Time spent away together intensifies your experiences. Making sex the focus of your break will revitalize your love life.

Bridget Jones turned the romantic "mini-break" into a joke, but if your relationship has been in a slump, a few days away is a perfect chance to recharge your sexual batteries.

Prioritizing sex rather than, say, sightseeing or dining, will fire up your love life for possibly months afterward. The reason is that a new place lets you reinvent yourselves. You'll be more daring and more focused on each other. And if you have any problem areas, you can plan to work them out over the weekend.

Here are some ideas for solving two common relationship problems during a typical two-day break. Use them as a model to write out your own "prescription for love." (Sorry, couldn't help myself.)

Here's an idea for you... **Get a room and experiment with those "pay-for-sex" fantasies that you've always meant to try together.**

Predicament: You're turning into "just good friends."
Goal: Reestablish yourselves as lovers.

It's oh-so-very easy to get into the rut of being good companions rather than red-hot lovers. Everything about your break should be geared to remind you of the sensual things in life. Don't make it about catching up on culture, unless you happen to get fantastically turned on by modern art. Think long, boozy lunches in shady cafes and then back to the hotel bed for a siesta because it's too damn hot to do much else. Think Spain or Italy.

The sexual focus of the weekend should be on rediscovering your excitement in each other and forging the bond between you as lovers. You could:

Day 1 Build excitement. Kiss, feel each other up, grope, spend hours on foreplay but break out of your rut by not having sex. Pretend that you are new lovers who aren't ready to move on to the sexual stage of a relationship. Be a little shy—shut the bathroom door. Take time with your appearance. See each other as you did in your first days together. Work on feelings of compassion and affection for your lover—see them through the same rose-colored specs that you did in the beginning. Be determined to find them deeply endearing, no matter how much they were irritating you yesterday. Allow yourself to be charmed.

Day 2 Resolve to do something you'll never forget. You can probably remember vivid details of your lovemaking during the first six months of your relationship. It's the last six years that are tricky. After the build-up of yesterday, create new shared memories of sex that will stay with both of you when you get home and fuel desire when the rut beckons again. Use the new location to the max. Move mirrors in your hotel room so that you can see yourselves while you have sex. Throw your lover against a wall in a tiny cobbled street. Slip away from the lights and do it on the beach.

Predicament: Your love life is predictable.
Goal: To regain the sparkle.

If getting away is a problem, try IDEA 51, *Fantasy destinations*.

Try another idea...

Usually when sex is predictable, you have temporarily lost that special feeling of closeness that gives you the confidence to initiate new things and explore your sexuality. Choose a location where it will be easy to relax and spend time talking with each other. Avoid anything that involves a lot of hassle or even excitement, so forget backpacking through Eastern Europe. Think quiet auberge in the South of France or luxurious English country house.

Day 1 Create intimacy. Turn your hotel bedroom into a sensual sanctuary. Take oils and candles from home. Spend a couple of hours bathing, showering, and massaging each other before dinner. Don't rush into sex (or if you do, maintain the sensual touching afterward). Live in the moment. Rediscover each other. Hold hands. Maintain eye contact as much as possible. Spend an hour talking about your feelings about work, family, friends, and your relationship. Your aim is to make your lover feel cherished and listened to.

Day 2 Break the patterns. Each write three things you'd like to try on a piece of paper. Think about this in advance so you have any props on hand. Take turns to fulfill each other's wishes. If you find this giving too hard, make it a game—be each other's sex slave.

"When you do something kinky, it's like, yes, the mango sex. We'll always remember the mango sex...It wasn't even that good, but we remember it. And that's the key—the remembering."
BETH LAPIDES, comedian

Defining idea...

How was
it for
you?

**Q   It's fine when we're away and for about a week afterward. Then
the lovey-dovey feelings go and it's back to business as usual.
How can we keep that lovin' feeling?**

A   *Make "change for change's sake" your mantra in every aspect of your life
together. It serves to make you more spontaneous with each other. For
instance, moving the position of your bed can subconsciously remind you to
keep things fresh in the bedroom. As can something as simple as swapping
sides of the bed. Who made the rule that he always sleeps on the left? Do
you always eat dinner at the table? Then have a picnic in front of the TV.
Does one of you take responsibility for cleaning the car? Then the other
one should do it for a month. If you're constantly making small subtle
changes in your everyday life, you'll automatically bring this into the
bedroom—or on the kitchen table if you're really entering into the spirit of
things. When change is an everyday part of your life, it's easier to suggest
something new sexually to your partner.*

Q   It's difficult for us to get time away. Are there any alternatives?

A   *Fine, just set aside two days together at home, and work out your timetable
of love. And if you really can't find the time to be at home together, you've
got a big problem. Very few people have reasons so genuine that they can't
find a way past them if they're motivated enough. If you're not motivated
enough, that's your problem. Talk about it first.*

16

Think kink

Remember: We don't always get what we want. But we can ask.

Your mission, should you choose to accept it, is to ask your partner to try something you're convinced has never occurred to them. This idea is a generic "how-to" on asking for this something, be it group sex, dogging, fisting, voting Republican, or whatever.

STATING THE OBVIOUS

If you want to try something out of the norm, then you'll have to communicate it to your lover either verbally or physically.

1. Butter them up first by faking a midlife crisis. Tell them you're worried that they'll leave you—couples are splitting up everywhere (give examples). Do this in a lighthearted way over a bottle of wine or in a worried way after faking moodiness that has them wondering what's wrong. I recommend the former,

but hey, it's your relationship. Tell them that although your love life is fine, you feel you've been complacent and you don't want them to get bored. Modify this basic script depending on your lover's gullibility levels but you get the basic idea—you make it your problem, not theirs. And then you make some changes to your love life.

2. Once you've mixed it up a little and you're regularly trying new things, suggest a modest first step on the way to what you want. If you want them to whip you with a cat of nine tails, then suggesting you experiment with a little mild pain via dripping candle wax is a good start.

3. Work up to the real deal. Be patient. Six months' patient if necessary.

Here's an idea for you...

If you're still shy about asking for what you really want, remember that the taboo of today is the norm of tomorrow. Rejoice in the thought of being a sexual pioneer, and pity all those guys who went through the '50s longing for a blow job but who were too afraid to ask in case they were thought to be perverts.

NEVER FORGET

The secret in persuading your lover to do something kinky that you want and they aren't particularly interested in is to make it clear that it's *them* doing the kinky thing that you're interested in, not the kinky thing itself. Use imagination, tact, and flattery to find a way to make this obvious.

Right: "Your butt looks amazing in rubber."
Wrong: "All I can think of is Michelle Pfeiffer in that Catwoman outfit."

Remember that the secret is *always* to make your lover feel special and to convince them how special they are to you. You'd be quite amazed at the things that some people can persuade others to do with this terribly simple strategy. But I've seen the police reports.

HOW NOT TO DO IT

I received a letter once from a man who couldn't understand why his new girlfriend wouldn't join him and his five best friends naked in a sauna for a beer. It turned him on so much and his ex-wife hadn't had a problem with it. Letting his friends leer at her and compare her with his previous girlfriend must have been an alluring prospect for the new girlfriend! He was clearly not as interested in women per se as in their willingness to get naked in front of his friends. Something told me that here was a man with a lot of disappointment ahead of him.

The last word: Most sex lives benefit from including a few of the minor elements from some of the major fetishes. So, give it a try and if it's not you, don't try it again.

Stuck for a kink to practice with? For inspiration turn to IDEA 21, *Bringing up the rear*, and IDEA 31, *Betty and Daisy rather than Sadie and Missy*.

Try another idea...

"[Kinky sex] is not about giving up 'normal' sex, adopting a new 'lifestyle.' joining a 'community,' or becoming a 'freak.' It's about making sex hotter. It's about giving voice to your darker, maybe even slightly disturbing desires by exploring new sensations, playing make-believe and other mind games. It's about making kink a part of your everyday sex life...OK maybe just your weekend and holiday sex life."
EM and LO, sex gurus on Nerve.com and authors of *The Big Bang*

Defining idea...

**Q   I want to get involved in group sex, just watching other couples.
I've mentioned it to my wife a few times, but she's not interested.
What's my next move?**

A   *I have little sympathy with the bullying lover—and I fear you're one. Sexual
bullies always play variations of this one theme: "I love my partner. I really
do. It's just always been my dearest sexual fantasy to watch group sex in a
parking lot and damn it, she just isn't interested." Sexual bullies always start
with "I love you" and end with "If you don't do it, I'll find someone else
who will." So, if you're heading in that direction, think carefully about what
that says about you.*

Q   When does kinky become a problem?

A   *If your lover starts expressing a wish for you to shave off your pubic hair,
walk on their back in stilettos, and stick Snickers bars up their butt, then
your job is to decide whether this is a lover who wants you to add some
spice to their sex life or whether the shaving, stilettos, and Snickers are an
absolute prerequisite to having good sex with you (or anyone else). If it's
the latter, you've got a fetishist on your hands and you have to decide
whether you want that fetish to be a constant factor in your love life. If you
can accept and incorporate your lover's kinks, they'll love you for it. I mean
really love you for it. There are few things more devoted than the fetishist
who is lucky enough to come across a lover who tolerates their obsession.
But if it's something you want only occasionally, you have to be strong
about your boundaries.*

17

Learn the art of kaizen

Kaizen is a Japanese concept that means "small changes, big differences." It can revolutionize your love life.

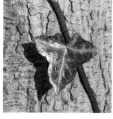

Psychologists say that if you want to keep dementia at bay you need to keep your brain on its toes. Your brain operates on well-worn grooves and you should break them to improve your chances of staying mentally alert.

You probably always brush your teeth in the way you perfected in childhood, but if you surprise your brain by brushing your teeth with the other hand, you'll force it to work harder and stay fresher. Changing your routine just slightly—taking a new route to work, kissing friends when you meet rather than hugging them, eating your main meal at noon—will give you a different perspective, a new way of looking at things. Mixing it up will do the same for your sex life.

Ban yourself from coming in your "normal" way for a month. You'll have to work harder for results, but you'll be forced to be more inventive.

Promise yourself that the next time you make love you will, as far as possible, work on the rule of difference. If you always start with kissing, try flipping your lover over and massaging their shoulders instead; if you prefer to be on top, then lie on your back; if you always come first, come second; if you almost always initiate sex, allow your lover to choose the time and place next time. You'll feel resistance, as your instincts will be to follow the same old pattern, but fight it. Let's cut to the chase: Absolutely nothing—infidelity, children, the clap—is more ruinous to your love life than having sex more or less the same way more or less all the time. Both of you need to try to make sex different every time you do it. Obviously not completely different, but just a little bit different from the last time or, better still, the half a dozen times before that. There are hundreds of different ways to stimulate your partner with your mouth and hands—try them. Or groan no if you always groan yes. Or grab a soft scarf and run it between your partner's legs before rubbing them through the material. Anything at all to reassure your partner that you're not operating on automatic pilot.

and another...

Look at every household object with renewed interest. Incorporate some of them into your lovemaking if possible— without frightening the neighbors.

Defining idea...

"It's OK to laugh in the bedroom so long as you don't point."
WILL DURST, satirist

As a rule of thumb:

1. Do something you haven't done in the last month or so every single time you make love.

2. Don't come in a certain position if you can remember exactly when you last came that way.

Turn to IDEA 30, *Assume the position*, for some ideas on jazzing up the "old faithful" positions.

Try another idea...

Q **The first and most important difference I'd like is for my wife to make the first move. If I wait for her to initiate sex, I'll wait forever. Why's that?**

How was it for you?

A *Check your own responses first. Has your wife ever kissed you, approached you for a cuddle, or held your hand when you just weren't in the mood? What did you do? Move away? Men often wish that their partner would initiate sex more, but what they really mean is initiate sex when they want it. Not, of course, when they're immersed in the game on TV, which would be annoying. And annoyed is what your wife feels when you leap on her while she's sorting laundry. Men are generally terrific at bouncing back from rejection because most tend to get lots of practice in adolescence, and they're also willing to put up with their partner taking a moment to get on their sexual wavelength. Women—much more thin-skinned—take that original hesitation on your part as outright rejection and turn away, perhaps for good. Be responsive when she's tactile, even if there's no* chance of it progressing to sex. Her reaching for your hand while you're shopping could be the beginning of foreplay that isn't consummated until after dinner. If you do all of the above and respond to every twitch of her affectionate nature, then you'll have to explain to her that always taking the initiative is making you feel like you're harassing her. Ask her to surprise you just once in the upcoming month. Don't pressure her and keep talking openly and gently.

Q   Isn't this kaizen exhausting?

A   If it's treated as a game, it's fun. More importantly, it will make you focus on your sexuality, and anytime you do that, your sex life will nearly always improve.

18

Building bridges

How can a woman come just like a man?

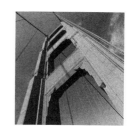

Women—if you could come as easily as your man, wouldn't you want to have sex more often? Men—if she came as easily as you did, wouldn't you be grateful?

A ton of foreplay is, of course, vital. Oral sex is, of course, important. Candlelit dinners, lots of chat, and making an effort for each other are critical for a long-standing, ever-loving relationship. But sometimes it's Monday night, you have an early start in the morning, you've had a long hard day, and you just want for both of you to come with the minimum of effort.

As the Hite Report—the most exhaustive description of female sexuality available—tells us, the great majority of women need clitoral stimulation with either hand or vibrator if they're going to come during penetrative sex. Still, the ideal persists that we should all be multiorgasmic by penile insertion. Frankly, it's bull. Thrusting the penis into the vagina is anatomically the same thing as pulling on a man's balls. You could make a man come eventually by this method—every tug would move the skin on the upper tip of the penis so eventually he might get enough stimulation—but boy, would it take a while. And for some men it would never work. The only hope for the vast majority of women is to get used to coming during penile penetration through clitoral stimulation.

Here's an idea for you...

Contract your vaginal muscles (PC muscles) as you approach orgasm. This will help bring on your orgasm and will also help you when you stop clitoral stimulation. Eventually, the contractions may be enough to power you into orgasm with no further clitoral stimulation. A few dirty words whispered in your ear won't hurt.

According to the irresistibly direct D. Claire Hutchins in her almost as irresistibly titled *5 Minutes to Orgasm: Every Time You Make Love*, "Millions of women enjoy orgasm during intercourse by using additional stimulation of the clitoris. The question should not be is this wrong? Can this be fixed? The question should be, why do we keep asking such a stupid question in the first place? Why resort to everything in the book, from scented candles and bubble baths, extensive analysis and sex therapy to make orgasm happen any other way. Ladies—let's move on. If the thought of touching yourself in front of your partner scares you, you'll have to get over it."

Bravo, D. Claire Hutchins. However, women and men do persist in feeling that they'd like to come from the same thrusting stimulation. And there is a way to do it: bridging. And what you're building is a "bridge" between clitoral and penile stimulation. The bridge maneuver means simply using clitoral stimulation—which most women need to orgasm—to bring the woman to the very edge of coming, then desisting and the woman coming following a few thrusts more from the man. This is a three-step process that anyone can learn, although it takes practice. Personally speaking, if you get to step two and come that way, you'll still be in a good place.

STEP 1: ADOPT THE POSITION

Find a position that allows maximum clitoral stimulation. It can be the missionary position or any other as long as your hand stimulates your clitoris. Best is the big mama of quick female orgasm: You straddle your partner, pull aside your labia and lean forward so that your clitoris rubs directly against his pelvic bone or sit upright so that you can masturbate your clitoris while on top of him.

If you have trouble knowing what to fantasize about (it happens!), turn to IDEA 50, Dream time.

Try another idea...

STEP 2: BRING YOUR MIND INTO PLAY

You're on top (or underneath, or hanging off the ceiling fan, whatever rocks your world), writhing about, touching yourself. Feel yourself getting closer to orgasm? No? OK, time to bring fantasy into the act. With fantasy, you stop worrying about your stomach jiggling, the kids' lost homework, whether he's getting bored or not, or whether you are. With fantasy, you concentrate on sex. With fantasy, you're the star of the show, the focus of the action—and you're gorgeous. Or as humorist Nora Ephron put it, "In my fantasy, no one loves me for my mind." Concentrate on achieving your orgasm. Shut your eyes. Forget about your man if necessary. Don't stop until you come, if you want to bridge...

STEP 3: BRIDGING

Take yourself to the very edge of orgasm and then stop the clitoral stimulation. Bring yourself off by grinding yourself against his body. This is partly a mental thing. When you believe you're going to come through penetration only, it's more likely that you will.

"Women can't alter the physiology in order to conform to what is expected of us, so we adopt countless strategies to reconcile reality with expectations, including faking orgasm. But who loses? Women do, and so do men. Instead of faking it, let's just accept our bodies and move on. Let's adjust."
D. CLAIRE HUTCHINS, writer

Defining idea...

79

How was it for you?

Q **I tried this but it hasn't worked yet. Any ideas?**

A *Masturbate more. Fine-tuning your sexual response by learning how to come as effectively as possible through masturbation is essential for most women wanting to come during penetration. If you do masturbate yourself to orgasm, then time yourself. How long from dead cold to orgasm? Between two to four minutes? Yup, that's normal. This is the average (just like men). If it's longer, keep practicing until you're under the four minutes. Then use this three-minute-something orgasm and experiment with the bridging techniques. Sorry if it sounds clinical and not very romantic. It is a little competitive, a little pressurized, and a little performance orientated. A bit like what sex is like for a guy, in fact. And that is the aim: To come efficiently and effectively every single time you have sex. Fabulous.*

Q **Why is masturbation such a big deal? Can't my man stimulate me?**

A *No, it's not about your man massaging you. Studies show that failure to orgasm is five times higher among women who never masturbate than among the rest of women; that out of approximately 10 percent of women who never orgasm, 95 percent have also never masturbated; that women who masturbate more come more often with their partners. I could go on...Just try it.*

19

When your sex drives are out of sync

Looking for a mate? Choose someone with roughly the same sex drive. Oh, sorry, you thought you had?

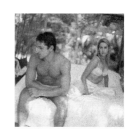

Every relationship goes through periods when one person wants sex more than the other—you're exhausted but your partner has one thing pretty obviously on their mind or vice versa.

ANY OF THE FOLLOWING FAMILIAR?

"I just don't want sex anymore"
This doesn't mean that you're always going to dread sex or that you won't regain your libido. There's nothing wrong with you either. What's far more likely is that your priorities have shifted and something else—job, kids, financial worries—is draining all your juice. Or it could be that for you sex is a demonstration of your closeness, but you feel distant from your partner: "We're miles apart, but he/she

Here's an idea for you...

The defining difference between couples having lots of sex and couples having virtually none is often a sense of playfulness. Play strip poker. Play Twister. Play doctors and nurses. Go to the movies and make out. Do anything that means you have fun and you'll almost inevitably rekindle passion.

still wants sex." If you're one of those people who, when single, always preferred having sex with someone you had a connection with, why would you change because you're in a long-term relationship? But as we all know, in a long-term relationship, you're not always completely in tune mentally with your partner.

Whether you're stressed or feeling distant, the solution is the same. Get closer. Talk to your partner and explain how you're feeling. Spend time holding each other. Create spaces in your life to do this. Switch the TV off and cuddle up in front of the fire. Go to bed half an hour earlier for "duvet time." Spend time being physically and emotionally close and eventually you'll want sex more often. It might not be great at first, but eventually you should reach a place where your libidos are more closely in sync again.

"My partner doesn't want me anymore"

Are you sure that this isn't more that they don't want sex at the same time as you? It's truly astonishing to me the number of men who report being hurt and resentful following repeated rejection from a wife who falls asleep by 9:30 most nights. Yet after a minute of careful questioning, it turns out they've never made the mental leap between her exhaustion and the fact that while he's lying in front of the TV, she's more often than not running around folding clothes, loading the dishwasher, or tidying up the day's debris. You have to be equally well rested for your libidos to get back in sync.

Don't hassle your partner for penetrative sex. Do hassle them for physical intimacy. You don't have the right to demand sex from your partner, but in a loving relationship, you are entitled to expect physical comfort and cherishing. And the latter makes the former a hell of a lot more likely. Increase physical intimacy, have just a little more sex, and wait out your partner's lost libido. With patience and (loving) perseverance, you can help them find it again.

Tiredness can be a passion killer, as can children. See IDEA 44, It's not all in your mind.

Try another idea...

"I am open to the guidance of synchronicity, and do not let expectations hinder my past."
DALAI LAMA

Defining idea...

How was it for you?

Q **It feels wrong to have sex when I don't enjoy it. What should I do?**

A *The most basic advice is to be sure to have an orgasm every time you make love. I'm prepared to bet that at the moment you're not. Masturbate after he comes (leave the bed if you're too shy, but think about why on earth you should be), buy a vibrator, or retrain your husband in a gentle way. Keep having sex, but make sure there's always a payback for you. Sure, sex can be great without an orgasm but it should happen on the minority, not the majority, of occasions. Otherwise, of course, you'll be bored and you're naturally going to resent him deep down somewhere.*

Q **I've tried being patient. We're doing lots of cuddling and kissing. We're also having a bit more sex, but although she seems to think it's enough, I want it to be the way it used to be for us. How can I recapture that?**

A *Time for honesty. Time for lateral thinking. Time to create new memories. Go away together. Stay at home together. Re-create your relationship from the bottom up. Pretend you're dating again. Be patient. If that doesn't work, seek professional counseling.*

20

What's your LQ score?

LQ = love quotient. What's yours?

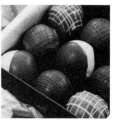

It's a weird one. Ten years into our relationship and we know more about what interests the person sitting next to us at work than the person we've chosen to share our lives with.

Years ago I read something in one of John Gray's books that has saved me a lot of grief since. John Gray wrote *Men Are from Mars, Women Are from Venus*, and the point he made—directed at men—was simple: If your partner adores chocolates and sees them as the eternal proof that you love her, why on earth would you buy her roses? Yet the world is full of guys turning up with bunches of roses and wondering why they get thrown at their head. The moral is simple: If your lover needs chocolates to make them feel loved, give 'em chocolates. It's irrelevant whether you think a bunch of red roses is more romantic. You need to give your partner what they need or you might as well not bother.

Here's an idea for you...

Feel your partner fails to listen to you? Sit him or her down and talk to him or her calmly. Huffing about or giving the silent treatment are passive-aggressive ways of getting nowhere. You have to spell it out.

Start looking for the "roses instead of chocolates" trait and you'll start seeing people everywhere doing loads for their loved ones that's going unnoticed. I was quite stunned to discover that after a make or break fight with my partner, all I had to do to appease him was cook him dinner. For whatever screwed up reasons of his psyche, what makes him feel loved isn't gifts of books, CDs, Thai prostitutes, or weekends away—it's me putting my apron on. And when I was upset with him, that's what he would do for me—cook me dinner. For a long time it got him nowhere, as what works for me when I feel angry is long extended conversations—and jewelry, of course. Jesting aside, it wasn't until I read the John Gray book that I got it. Our LQs were low. But now when I need to butter him up I just throw a steak on the grill. And when he's upset me, he grits his teeth and gets prepared to bare his soul.

Broadly speaking, to successfully love the person we're with we need to understand what they need to feel loved. To keep their love we must give them what they need as far as possible. If you're reading this and wondering what this has to do with sex, my answer to you is, "Duh! Just about everything." Lots of couples are having indifferent or absolutely no sex, not because they don't spark off each other but because they haven't felt loved by their partner for years. The classic example is the man faced with a distraught wife, who will do something practical for her—put up shelves, clean her car, pay the bills—when all she wants is a babysitter booked and a meal out.

When your lover's feeling insecure, stressed, or worried, how do you make them feel safe and reassured? Does it work? If not, do you know what would? If yes, why do you withhold it from them? Do you like to play mean just for the hell of it? It might seem to work and it might keep you the "superior" partner, but the price is high. Your partner won't be able to trust you and that sort of trust is essential to keep sex hot between you when the first thrill has gone.

Getting close physically in a non-sexual way inevitably makes it easier to get closer emotionally. Try IDEA 1, *Stop having sex.*

Try another idea...

Would your lover rather have a romantic meal or a wild night out on the town as a prelude to sex? Do you occasionally indulge them, even if you'd rather do something else?

"Sex is a conversation carried out by another means."
PETER USTINOV

Defining idea...

Does your partner feel closer to you when you're laughing together or being upset with you? If the answer's "upset," do you respond in a way that seems to satisfy them or are they disappointed in you? If the answer's "laughing," when was the last time you went out of your way to make sure you had a good laugh together?

What's your lover's favorite way of resolving a fight (not necessarily the way you always resolve it)?

These are the kind of questions you have to know the answers to. And your partner, of course, has to know what works for you. Emotionally we have to be given chocolates at least some of the time or we start to shut off from our partner and get tempted by someone who appears to offer Godiva on demand. If you're with someone for whom chocolate equals love, all the roses in the world won't fix your relationship or help you get good sex.

How was it for you?

Q **We get along fine without having to analyze each other too closely. Why start?**

A *Great. Hope it lasts. But one of the routes to a dull relationship is losing touch with your partner's inner life. Couples need a common goal or they stagnate. Even if you hate analyzing each other (or more likely, one of you hates it and imposes that on the other), at least once yearly shoot the breeze about what you want from the next twelve months. What would you like to experience? Visit? Achieve? Is there anything in common that you can work on together?*

Q **My partner won't share anything. How can I change the situation?**

A *When you're distant, a shortcut to getting on better is simply to act as if your relationship is perfect—if your lover never speaks to you, continue talking to them as if they're the world's greatest listener; if your lover never spontaneously shows affection, continue hugging. Sounds crazy, but the change from negative to positive somehow seeps through to your partner at least long enough for you to ask them to behave more lovingly and for them to hear what you're saying. Keep asking to share, but if they won't it's counseling for you, I'm afraid. Or you could just put up with it and find some mate with the emotional depth you crave. I still maintain it'll be hell on your long-term sex life though.*

21

Bringing up the rear

Sorry, terrible pun, but the alternative was "bottoms up," so consider yourself lucky.

Just twenty years ago, anal sex was shocking and unmentionable, but now you can switch on the TV and hear references to it quite routinely. But even if it wasn't talked about much, rear entry has always been mainstream—it's the original form of birth control.

Many couples try anal sex in the first lust-fueled months of their relationship and then forget about it. If you've tried it and your attitude is "Been there, done that, don't know what the fuss is about," then it might be time to revisit it. It can add a definite embellishment to your lovemaking.

Here's an idea for you...

It goes without saying that a bath or shower together is always a good idea before any sort of rear action. Clip your nails.

NO LONGER RISQUÉ, JUST PLAIN RISKY

Since you're reading this book, chances are you are already a "fluid bonded" couple, but if not then you need to practice safe sex. Plus, if you touch the anus with tongue, finger, dildo, or vibrator, you don't move forward without giving it a good cleaning. That isn't me making judgments—it's sheer common sense. Bacteria from the cleanest anus can still produce a fearful vaginal infection.

Violet Blue, a sex trainer, has a good tip if you hate interrupting sex to get safe. Wear some rubber gloves and condoms for anal play before peeling them off for vaginal intercourse.

WHY DO SO MANY MEN FANTASIZE ABOUT DOING IT?

I asked some men and their responses included:

■ "It makes me feel in control and powerful."

■ "She only agrees to it when she's really horny and sometimes I set myself the challenge of getting her so turned on that she wants it."

■ "It feels different, tighter. Some of my friends say it doesn't, but it does for me."

And let's not forget the latent homosexual element either, eh, boys?

BUT WHAT'S IN IT FOR WOMEN?

Embarrassed to ask? Turn to IDEA 16, *Think kink*.

Try another idea...

Anal sex for men causes friction against the prostate gland—a wonderful thing I'm told, although I'm not qualified to say. But what about for women? The vulval area responds to stretching and that sense of being filled up is terrific for most women. Anal sex works in the same way. Tongues, fingers, dildos, and butt plugs can all drive both sexes wild because they give the contracting orgasmic muscles in the butt something to work against.

Lubrication

It's only in porn films that saliva and free-flowing love juices provide enough lubrication to really enjoy anal sex. That's not to say it can't be done. Half a pint of tequila taken orally is a pretty good lubrication, too, I find. This brings me to another good point. You don't want to be numb when you're having anal sex— from alcohol or from those lubricants sold in sex shops that contain numbing ingredients under the mistaken impression that it's a good thing not to feel sore. Pain is a sign that your body should desist from what it's doing. Anal sex shouldn't be painful and if it is you need to stop and figure out what you're doing wrong.

Rimming

Lots of nerve endings on the anus means that the tongue put to good use can be almost as enjoyable as receiving oral sex. If it doesn't give you an orgasm, it can tip you right over the edge into one. Most common is to use your tongue held at a point to circle around the anal

"If everything was coated with a seal of approval, some of the fun would go out of it. Let's get away with something. Degrade me, baby."
SALLY TISDALE, writer

Defining idea...

opening and penetrate in and out, but start with a loose tongue—big licks along the crack feel great and loosen everyone up. Some people like nibbles along the length working toward the anus. As ever, don't put your tongue anywhere else until you've rinsed your mouth.

Penetration

Don't attempt anal penetration until your partner is well and truly revved up and a ton of lubrication has been used. Press your finger against the anus, applying pressure.

Massage the opening and slowly slide your finger in up to the first joint. Stay still. You'll feel the ring of muscles around the anus tighten and relax. Don't move your finger, just let the muscles work. When they relax again, slide your finger in slowly.

For women: Men can experiment with a finger in the anus and a thumb in the vagina.

For men: Women can stimulate his prostate, but only when he's truly aroused. You'll feel it as a nub on the front wall of the anus a couple of inches in. It gets bigger as a man gets older and is often described as being the size of a walnut. It responds to pressure and stroking—don't poke and don't prod. Depending on the man this can be quite firm stroking or rhythmic pressure. Ask him for feedback. Stimulation of the prostate while using your mouth or hand to massage his penis results, apparently, in a dynamic, deep orgasm.

Once you've tried with a finger, the world's your oyster. There's a joke there somewhere, but I don't want to think about it too much. If penetrating with a penis or a dildo, the same applies—gentle, rubbing action, unless your lover tells you different, and slow penetration.

Q **I like anal sex and I'd like to try introducing some toys. Literally. It's safe enough, isn't it?**

How was it for you?

A *For my sins I know a lot of doctors and one of the common after-dinner conversations when doctors meet socially is recalling the different objects they've had to extricate from patients' butts. There's a book to be written here, but you'll be relieved to hear this isn't it. Be careful: Never insert anything that isn't smooth, unbreakable, and flared at the bottom.*

Q **Such as?**

A *Butt plugs provide a terrific sense of fullness and make contractions during orgasm more intense. Holding a vibrator against the butt plug gives delicious sensations. Those small bullet vibrators are almost sitting up and begging to be stuck up your butt, but caution brothers and sisters: Most sex toys are shoddily made. Relying on yanking out a bullet or anything else by the electric wire is likely to leave you holding a bit of wire and with a big problem. Stick to rubbing bullets on the perineum.*

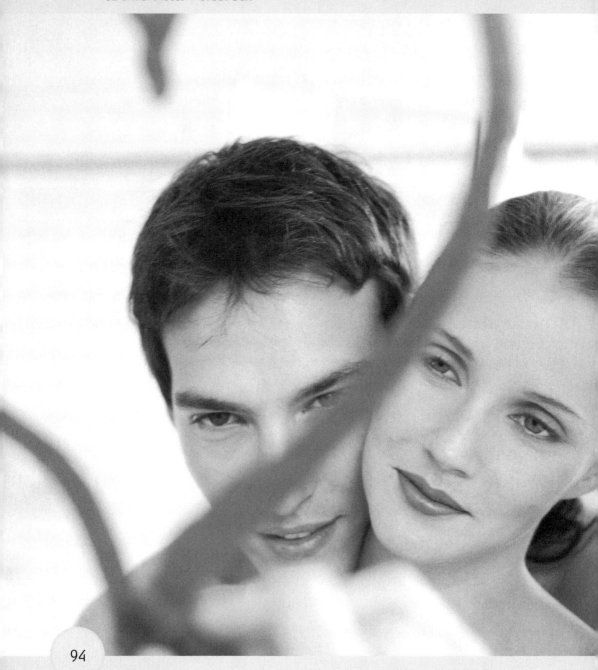

22

Sexual confidence

What is sexual confidence? And how can you get your hands on some?

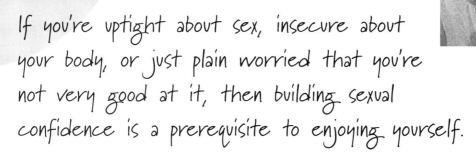

If you're uptight about sex, insecure about your body, or just plain worried that you're not very good at it, then building sexual confidence is a prerequisite to enjoying yourself.

What factor most affects your ability to have a wonderful sex life? A great body? A fabulous lover? A bendy body? If you've got all these, good for you. Even so, without one all-important element, your sex life is still likely to be ho-hum rather than fantastic. You must have sexual confidence.

WHAT MIGHT WORK

This is where my feminist principles go out of the window. Truth is, if you're feeling lackluster about your appearance—male or female—it's very unlikely you're having a great sex life. Time to lose the weight. A dramatic weight loss in a long-term partner should always be viewed with terrific suspicion. If your lover loses pounds and your love life is less than sparkling, you'd better start improving your bedroom skills because their sexual confidence is going to go sky high and when that happens, thrilling sex is never far away. With or without you.

Here's an idea for you... **Work on feeling more sexual every day. Think of yourself as a powerfully sexual person. Look for opportunities to make life more sensual. Flirt.**

On the other hand, if you've been feeling less like sex, ask yourself whether being five pounds lighter would make a difference to your libido. If it would, then diet.

And this is where I go the whole nine yards and tear up my ticket as a card-carrying feminist. I would love to write with bravado that if you think having bigger/firmer/smaller boobs would improve your sex life you're crazy. But I'm not sure. As a child, I smashed my teeth falling off a bike. I had bad veneers fitted to replace them. As I proceeded through my twenties, I became self-conscious about smiling and eventually even about talking, so I had new, more expensive dental work and felt more confident. Do I have the right to sneer at those who think fiddling with their body parts will make a difference to their sexual confidence? No. But beware. Your goal is sexual confidence. If it's your partner who wants you to have surgery, you won't gain sexual confidence. And if you've had a boob job already, I very much doubt that having smoother thighs will make the difference. These are distractions, and your relationship with either your partner or yourself is at fault. Spend your money on therapy or a self-esteem course instead.

Finally, if you're a man, please don't waste your money on penis-enhancing aids that you see in magazines. I'd like to say to you that women don't worry about size, but I can't, because they do. But it would be an unusual woman who ditched a guy because his penis didn't live up to her previous lover's penis. If your penis is smaller than average—anything less than five inches erect—you'll have to be kinder, smarter, funnier, and better in bed than other men. Unfair, I know, but life isn't fair.

Some penis pumps will work temporarily. There are apparently two operations that can increase either the girth or the length of the penis that actually work. They also can cause problems, and if the penis-lengthening operation goes wrong, you actually end up with a shorter penis. I jest not.

Feeling cherished can do wonders for our sexual confidence. For ways to do this for your lover look at IDEA 13, Touchy-feely.

Try another idea...

SO WHAT DOES WORK?

- **Change your perception.** Do what it takes for you to feel as attractive as you can. Then start talking yourself up: "I'm happy," "I look great," "I'm gorgeous." Repeat your affirmations twenty times daily.

- **Look in a mirror.** As we get older or busier, we spend less time looking in the mirror and try to pretend our body just isn't there. A mistake. Buy a full-length mirror. Look at yourself naked. Look at yourself dressed. Spend time preening. Throw out everything that doesn't make you feel and look great. If that leaves you with three items of clothing, so be it.

- **Spend as much time as you can naked.** This reacquaints you with your body and puts you in touch with your sexual self.

"If you're one of those people who can't even look in the mirror naked, you need to get used to it. Maybe you need to start with underwear. Maybe you need to start with a parka, and work down from there. The point is...you're going to have to get comfortable in your own skin."
DR. PHIL MCGRAW, writing in *O Magazine*

Defining idea...

■ **Devote an hour a week to loving your body.** If pampering isn't you, start exercising or go to a massage therapist or reflexologist. Anything that gets you back in touch with that thing you need for sex—your body.

How was it for you?

Q   I need to lose weight, but I just can't. What'll make me succeed?

A   *If you were thinner, how would you behave? What would you be doing? Exercising, eating healthily, buying nice clothes? OK. How can you start doing that tomorrow? The mistake most would-be dieters make is to think in abstract rather than concrete terms and be too ambitious. You can start exercising tomorrow, but it's highly unlikely you'll start jogging around the park four days a week, which is probably the unrealistic goal you've set for yourself. It's also highly unlikely you're going to give up chocolate and chips overnight, but you could aim to eat fruit or vegetables at every meal. You could buy yourself one nice item of clothing, even if it's in a bigger size—it will make you feel better about yourself. Build up until you're following the sort of lifestyle that will mean you reach your goals.*

Q   I find my partner less attractive since he got fat. He keeps saying he'll do something about it, but his attempts last two days max. Am I being unreasonable?

A   *Your attitude is just the sort that won't help. Research studies have shown that it takes people many attempts to succeed at reaching a weight goal, but if they keep persevering, they'll get there. One of the factors that helps them is the unwavering, nonjudgmental support of family. That's you.*

23

What you see...

The general consensus is that men get turned on more than women by visual stimulation. But is it true?

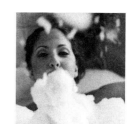

Could it be that women, freed up to be more sexual, are just beginning to find out what turns them on visually?

The writer J. K. Collins, who was the advice columnist in the first soft porn magazine aimed at heterosexual women, *For Women*, wrote an interesting book entitled *The Sex We Want*. One of the points she makes is that we know a lot about what men find sexually stimulating, but nothing much about what works for women.

I think this applies to visual stimulation in particular. When they view porn, even lousy misogynistic porn, women get sexually aroused in just the same physiological ways as men, i.e., there's a flood of blood to their sexual organs. What would the result be of watching porn aimed at exciting both men and women? My point is that women may be able to use visual stimulation to turn them on just as regularly and efficiently as men use it.

During a research group into young women's sexuality that I led for a publishing house, one of the women in the group confessed that she would turn herself on by

Here's an idea for you... **Check out your local large bookstore's erotica section— they've improved in terms of both quality and quantity in the last couple of years.**

pretending to be a stripper in front of a mirror in her bedroom. She really was a private dancer as she cheerfully admitted she would be too embarrassed to perform a striptease for her boyfriend, but she loved to watch while she gradually dropped her clothes until she was naked.

I was reminded of her when I read this passage from *The Hite Report*, where a woman describes how she masturbates: "Sometimes I dress in erotic costumes and view myself in the mirror. Usually I smoke a cigarette and sometimes I put on makeup. If there is time, I lubricate my breasts and genitals with oil or cream. I prefer looking in the mirror rather than directly at myself. I begin playing with my breasts..."

Another woman in *The Hite Report* says, "My best 'quickie, one-minute special' is standing up with my vibrator, on my toes, totally tensed...with the vibrator tip against the clitoris and holding the body of the vibrator out, so it looks like a penis— in front of the mirror. I get turned on by my image doing this and come in a minute."

What's interesting is that all these women observe themselves. Is that for want of any other material? My theory is that once women get used to the idea of getting turned on visually, they will. As J. K. Collins points out in her book, the failure of sex magazines aimed at women (including *For Women*) could have something to do with the fact that they can't show erect dicks. (When you think about what's out there now, how ridiculous is that?) Still, women might find that gay magazines aimed at either sex work for them. Or it could be the sight of restraints on your lover. Or dressing him as a gladiator. Actively look for images that turn you on and use them in fantasy and lovemaking to make you feel more sexually vibrant. The reason I think this is worth going on about is that it's one of the easiest and quickest ways to keep your libido alive and kicking, and we need as much of that as we can in a long-term relationship.

Turn to IDEA 48, *See things differently*, for other ways of exploring visual stimulation.

Try another idea...

Wear clothes to bed that turn you on. If you love the way your breasts look in a push-up bra, keep it on. I know one woman who wore a favorite pair of red stilettos to bed. They did nothing for her man, but she used to lie with her feet in the air, admiring what those shoes did for the length of her legs. Love yourself!

This is all easier for women as the sexual female body is a ubiquitous image (and why women find it easy to observe themselves for titillation), but men don't often get the chance to be sex objects. So why not be different? If you really want to rock her world, rent a fireman's outfit for the night. I have no idea why, but it would be a rare woman who wouldn't appreciate the gesture.

Use mirrors—line them up so you can see yourself from all angles. Then experiment with lighting. A flashlight adds a creepy, otherworldly quality to proceedings and you might find that interesting. It's also hard to get the image of having sex by candlelight out of your mind afterward, which is a bit less scary and a lot more flattering than a camcorder. Though of course, that works on the same principle.

"Sexual intercourse is kicking death in the ass while singing."
CHARLES BUKOWSKI, writer

Defining idea...

How was it for you?

Q   Books, films, etc., don't do a thing for me. What's my next move?

A   OK. But remember, it's just conditioning that tells men that garters and stockings are sexy. A friend of mine spent months mincing around the bedroom in various versions of the full outfit, with no significant effect on her boyfriend. She finally asked him what turned him on (radical idea, I know) and he answered, "One of those neck to floor white cotton nightdresses like your granny might wear, with buttons up the front." Who would have ever guessed? You may have to be sexual commandos, fearlessly tracking down new territory before you find what turns each other on.

Q   Any suggestions for women-friendly visual aids?

A   Try the web: www.nerve.com has a photo gallery, or there's the bookstore at www.gash.co.uk. You could also try making your own porn movie (turning the camcorder on you and your lover, I hasten to add). Reliving some of your greatest moments before you get it on should spur you onto greater heights.

24

Blow jobs 101

Put a little thought into your next blow job—he'll appreciate it.

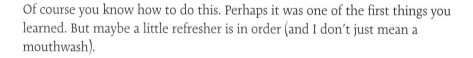

Boy meets girl. Girl meets boy. Love and mutual respect blossoms. And before long the question of fellatio raises its occasionally ugly head.

Of course you know how to do this. Perhaps it was one of the first things you learned. But maybe a little refresher is in order (and I don't just mean a mouthwash).

THE BASIC MENU

Whatever your technique, it's worth making sure it includes these moves:

- Use your tongue to circle around the rim on the head of the penis quite firmly and to run up and down the ridge on the underside until it meets the small piece of skin where the head meets the shaft—the frenulum. Doing this stimulates two of the most sensitive parts of the penis (if he's uncircumcised—but try it even if he is).

Here's an idea for you...

Ask him to run his hands through your hair or touch the side of your face while you're going down on him. Men don't often think to do this, and women don't ask them because for most women the sense of having their head controlled is an unpleasant one, but there's a world of difference between a man keeping contact by gently ruffling your hair and gripping your ears in a death grip.

Defining idea...

"Oral sex is currently very trendy. It is even preferred to the regular kind. It is preferred because it's the only way most of us can get our partners to shut up."
P. J. O'ROURKE

■ Massage the perineum (the spot between the testicles and anus) while you're going down—a vibrator is good for this.

■ After years together, you may be taking his pleasure somewhat for granted. For most men, the easiest way to make them think they're getting a great blow job is for you to seem to be having a good time. So, give it all the enthusiasm you would the finest chocolate ice cream and if the odd moan of pleasure escapes all the better. Or you could hum—some women swear by humming while they're giving oral sex, as the vibrations heighten the sensation on the penis.

EXTRAS

Add sensations that make him even more aware of what's going on down there.

1. Swirl mouthwash around your mouth before going down. The mint tingles and makes him more tuned in to the heat of your mouth. Toothpaste gives an even more extreme sensation.

2. Bite into a lemon.

3. Hold a mouthful of neat vodka in your mouth as long as you can. Try this tentatively at first. Sensitive souls feel it as a burn.

Turn to IDEA 33, *More on blow jobs*, for more ideas on giving him oral sex.

Try another idea...

4. Hot tea (not boiling) used the same way can engulf him in a warm bath of sensation.

5. An ice cube crushed in your mouth will be excruciatingly sensitive. Or keep the ice cube intact and work it around his penis as you move your mouth up and down.

6. If you're really coordinated, try hot and cold in succession. This can be quite a feat, so to keep him in sexual wonderland and retain your mystique it helps to blindfold him first, kiss him generously all over, fool him that that's the main course, and then make with the hot/cold routine. Done teasingly this can be great fun for both of you.

"Fellating is fun, but it's hard work. After twenty minutes it's just hard work."
EM and LO, sex columnists on Nerve.com

Defining idea...

How was it for you?

Q **I've tried your tips, but my partner is pretty silent and I don't know if he's embarrassed by the moves or enjoying them. How can I find out?**

A   *You need to make it clear in a charming way to your partner that staying silent when receiving oral sex isn't helpful. Appreciative groans are the very least that a lover should expect. It's good manners and it spurs you on to greater efforts. But better than muttering is clear direction. We are probably more individualistic in the way we prefer to receive oral sex than anything else in the sexual repertoire. One woman I interviewed told me that her husband preferred her to use her teeth—hard—when she was going down on him. Now this is unusual, and my point is not to start gnawing on your lover's manhood (although some men may well enjoy a light grazing). My point is that you don't know what he likes unless he tells you. Even if it's a long-standing partner, ask. Take the pressure off him by making it non-judgmental on your performance. It helps to say, "Do you like this (demonstration) better than this (further demonstration)?" Most times the response will be "Whatever, just don't stop." But occasionally you'll learn something useful.*

Q   **It takes ages for me to come. What's the best route to home base?**

A   *Give her a break and change the rhythm—use your hand or encourage her to swap to penetration or hand jobs. If she's just not giving you the right stimulation, vary your technique. Do you find it hard to relax and enjoy oral sex? This is common in women and there's no reason why men should escape. Women do like fellating and can really get off on it. Talk to your lover and perhaps use fantasy to overcome an inability to relax.*

106

25

Dressing up and staying in

Acting out fantasies takes some practice but can certainly brighten up a boring Saturday night.

First get into bed and talk dirty to each other. Read from some mildly pornographic books (or filthy pornographic books, if you like). Share some situations that turn you on mentally. Talk through the sorts of things you'd like to say or do.

The next obvious step is to pick a night to play out your fantasy, although sometimes it's best just to go for it spontaneously, as it helps you to feel less self-conscious. Even if the first time is a disaster and lasts about two minutes before you start laughing, at least you've started.

You won't have to expend any money on special outfits unless you want to, as you can improvize with dressing up and props. Again, it helps if one of you (the one who will be dominant in the fantasy makes the most sense) takes control of organizing and briefing the other on their role.

Here's an idea for you... **Crack open a bottle (or two). As with all fantasy games, alcohol helps loosen you up. A lot.**

Some people find costumes liberating and that they help them get into character. Some people find them inhibiting, not to say ridiculous. But don't give up on them too early because they can help. Before you know it, you'll be down at the local costume shop for your Robin Hood or nun's outfit.

SIX CLICHÉD (AND-THAT'S-BECAUSE-THEY-WORK) FANTASY ROLE-PLAYS

Doctor and nurse

It's the end of another grueling day on the wards. The nurse (either one of you) is looking exhausted. The doctor calls the nurse over and says, "You're looking tired. Need a complete examination?" The doctor gets the examination table ready and asks the nurse to lie down on it. A complete physical later and the diagnosis is "nervous tension." However, the doctor is conducting a scientific study into this condition, with some controversial treatment options. If the nurse is willing to take part in some medical experimentation and give feedback on how well the cure works, the doctor will demonstrate the technique…

Master and slave

One of you is the cruel master (or mistress); one is the gorgeous slave. The master is deciding whether to buy or not, which involves a thorough examination. The slave is wrapped in layers of clothes but is slowly stripped (or ordered to strip) so the master can confirm that the slave is in good physical condition—and that means that every bit of them is in good physical condition. Then, of course, the slave's ability to follow orders and please the master will have to be tested…

Boss and interviewee

The interviewee comes to the office after hours to be interviewed for their dream job. The interview starts normally: The interviewee is anxious to please and the interviewer is gracious. However, when they start discussing terms of employment, some of the terms are quite unusual. Late-night working? Threesomes with the head of personnel and the boss? Finally, there is an initiative test—how well the interviewee performs determines whether they get the job...

Husband and the Swedish au pair

He is the innocent, she the fun-loving au pair (extra points if she can keep the accent going all the way through). The wife is away and he's settling down to watch football when she asks if she can join him. Is he seeing things or is her skirt always that short? And is she sitting a little closer than normal? She seems more flirtatious, more brazen. Double meanings and loaded looks are passing between them. He tries to get a grip on himself and resist temptation while she goes out of her way to seduce him into making the first move. Until finally, losing patience, she makes her intentions quite clear...

IDEA 50, *Dream time*, has more on fantasy.

Try another idea...

"It would be rude to get your sexual satisfaction by tying someone to the bed and then leaving him or her there and going out with someone more attractive."
P. J. O'ROURKE

Defining idea...

Handyman and housewife

He arrives ready for work, but she insists he has a cup of coffee first. While she's showing him the problem "with her pipes," she gets into such a position that he can't help noticing she's not wearing any underwear...

Naughty maid and "master of the house"

She's supposed to be cleaning the house when the "master" comes home and discovers her pleasuring herself instead. He's furious and threatens her with dismissal. She is beside herself. She'll lose her job. She has to think of something quick that will persuade him that sacking her is a bad idea...

Q **I think about acting out fantasies, but I feel too self-conscious. How can I get over this?**

How was it for you?

A *Acting out a role that's already predetermined removes performance pressure, so copy some scenes from movies. You'll then have a rough dialogue already—what you can remember from the script. For instance, anyone can do a bad Scottish accent and an unbelievable Eastern European one, so every couple can play James Bond and Bond Girl. A couple I know of used to be Jessica Lange and Jack Nicholson in* The Postman Always Rings Twice. *It was their shorthand for wild out-of-control sex and whenever she wanted some, he'd come home to find her roaming about their kitchen sporting low cleavage, tight skirt, extremely high heels, and a drawl like Blanche Dubois on a pint of bourbon. In his words, "I wanted her so much, I couldn't walk straight." After a bit of flirting, he'd throw her on the kitchen table and rip her clothes off.*

Q **Our home doesn't lend itself to acting out fantasies. How can we set the scene?**

A *Lighting helps. Make sure that you have low-key lighting, whether from candles, a flashlight, or a low lamp—whatever is appropriate for the fantasy. But please, this doesn't have to be an Oscar-winning production. The main thing is to get rid of any clutter—especially the kids' toys and any photos of your mother. The only essential in terms of location is to get rid of anything that even the world's most active imagination would balk at finding sexy.*

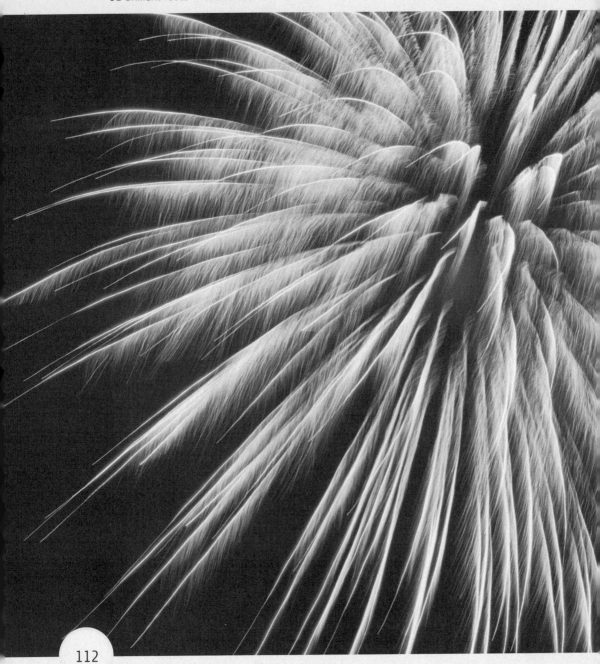

26

Handy work

What they never taught you in art class.

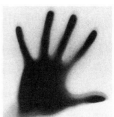

Getting your partner off with your hand is a staple of a good sex life and for men an essential skill to develop, as this is the only way most women can come during intercourse.

We get into habits with achieving orgasm, just like everything else. We are welded to one way of stimulating ourselves to climax and then (if we're lucky) our partners get proficient at mimicking us and that's the sort of stimulation we get from them. Terrific. No one's knocking that, but changing it up and using a different technique can teach you a lot about your sexual response and can result in deeper orgasms. It starts off as a frustrating process—it takes a while to retrain yourself—but rely on the Tantric principle, "It's the journey not the arrival that's important." Doing this will make you closer as a couple and it will make you more orgasmic.

Experiment with the following techniques when you're masturbating—once you've got the hang of them, share your new knowledge with your partner. Remember, if you're the one doing the stimulating, don't change between techniques too much in one session, as it's distracting, especially when your partner's approaching orgasm.

Here's an idea for you...

Lots of manual work can lead to chafing, so lubricate, lubricate, lubricate. Then lubricate some more.

DIFFERENT FOR GIRLS

■ Make a fist, place it on the top of the vulva and move it from there. Experiment with position and pressure until you find what works best. Careful, because it's easy to ruin the mood by being too enthusiastic—this one needs lots of communication.

■ After rubbing the clitoral area with fingers, moving onto a palm provides an intense pressure and an intense orgasm. Using the heel of the palm to grind against the clitoris while the fingers are free to play around with the vagina, perineum, and labia gives strong contractions, especially if you press down just above the pubic bone at the same time with your other hand. If you're doing this to your partner, it works well in positions where she is free to grind against the heel of your palm.

■ The wishbone, sometimes known as "the V," uses the whole of the clitoris and not just the little nub that we call the clitoris—that's just the part we see. Spreading outward and downward from the clitoris nub, on either side of the vagina and under the skin, are the arms of the clitoris. Place your index and middle fingers pointed downward toward the vagina, one on each side of the labia with the junction of the V on your clitoris nub. Massage the clitoral arms and the clitoris with the V, keeping up constant pressure on all parts of the clitoris. The orgasm from this technique takes time, but that builds tension and gives most women a more diffuse orgasm that's more of a whole body experience. Partners can use this during rear-entry positions by reaching around your waist.

- Insert the index finger of one hand into the vagina and push down very gently (if you're masturbating, reaching from behind with your hand might be easier). With the other finger rub up and down on the clitoral hood. The stretching will feel great.

Women: For explosive orgasms combine manual work with IDEA 29, Easy routes to faster orgasms for her.

Try another idea...

MEN ONLY

- After some preliminary strokes to get things heated up, hold the penis with one hand and place the palm of the other hand across the head. For every up movement and down movement, circle the other hand over the head. As one hand comes up you circle over. As the hand goes down you circle again. The hands come close together on the up stroke. Get into a rhythm.

- Clasp both hands around the penis with fingers interlaced and move up and down.

- Make your hands into two "beaks." Use one starting at the base of the penis and move up and another around the balls and pull them slightly outward at the same time. Relax. Repeat. This takes practice and isn't enough to get most men off, but it's terrific for men who like their balls played with.

"I don't say anything during sex. I've been told not to. Told during sex, in fact."
CHEVY CHASE

Defining idea...

115

■ Here's one to practice as he's approaching orgasm. Clasp both hands around the head of his penis and squeeze, hold for a second, let go, and squeeze again. You're trying to mimic the rhythm of his pulse and it can heighten the orgasm if done while he's ejaculating.

How was it for you?

Q   My partner says I'm too rough. Do you have any guidelines?

A   *Men: If you're not sure about how much pressure to apply and what rhythm to adopt when you're getting a woman off with your hand, the general advice is to go half as hard and twice as slow as you think will work. Get feedback from your partner. Encourage her to let you know when she wants it done differently. As with oral sex, if she's bucking against your hand that's a good indication that she likes what you're doing and wants harder, faster stimulation.*

Q   I come when I masturbate, but not when my husband uses his hand, even though he's doing it right. What's wrong?

A   *It could be that you have a mental block with this for some reason. Use fantasy to get over it. You're taking part in a medical experiment—the results will save humankind. You're a goddess and your high priest's greatest pleasure is servicing you. Orgasm is a mind game so cheat your brain.*

27

Heading south

Enjoy the journey and she'll be ecstatic.

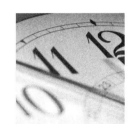

It's been said that if you think of the clitoris as being the center of a clock, most women get the most pleasure at 10 to 2. Want to know more? Then read on.

"When a lover goes down on me, anything can happen. From the first silky caress of a warm tongue on my clitoris to the crashing moment of orgasm as a hot mouth envelopes my vulva, I have the possibilities of the world between my legs. I can be anyone, anywhere: a woman arrested for speeding, bent over the hood of her car...I can role-play with my lover as a ravished femme, a dominant mistress, or a naughty schoolgirl. I can be the one woman my partner desires the most, with their face deliciously pressed between my legs in an act of worship that I can enjoy as either sacred or profane. But whenever, however, wherever it happens, I know I'm going to have a sexual experience that is at once tender and intimate, one that results in a powerful, focused orgasm."

That's how Violet Blue, a sex instructor, starts her book *The Ultimate Guide to Cunnilingus*, and I quote it in full because it reminds us why going down is tops. It guarantees an orgasm for more women, more of the time. Women who find it difficult to come find it easy this way.

Here's an idea for you...

This one comes from Violet Blue's *Ultimate Guide to Cunnilingus*. **Make a diamond with your hands and lay this over the labia to hold the "lips" apart to give you full access. Leaning against the bridge made by your fingers also gives you support when you need it.**

Defining idea...

"Porn is a lousy place to learn how to perform oral sex on a woman: most on-screen cunnilingus looks like an exaggerated version of Fido with a mouthful of peanut butter. However, adult instructional videos can be very helpful."
VIOLET BLUE, sex instructor

POSITIONS

Three things are essential:

1. The woman should be able to relax and not worry about supporting herself, such as lying back on the bed or sitting on the edge of a table.

2. The man should be comfortable—he might be there for a while. If you're on a bed, then support her butt on a couple of pillows. Or she could lie with her legs over the edge of the bed and he can kneel on the floor. Or do a variation of this on any table, chair, tabletop, etc.

3. Some couples enjoy the classic subservient oral sex pose. Men, you're the subservient one—on your knees while she stands in front of you. But this can make access difficult for you, and orgasm difficult for her. It's a bit easier if she supports one leg on a chair or low table, but the biggest thrill from this one tends to be the dominatrix element, not the position.

Men: 69s are fun and so is the traditional "sitting on the face" position. These look great visually—which is why they're so popular in porn films—as well as being exciting and/or

Read more on cunnilingus in IDEA 32, *Heading even farther south.*

Try another idea...

relaxing for you. But just so you know, although women can get deeply excited during these positions, few women will go over the edge and come. That's because women tend to have to be able to relax and concentrate in the buildup to their orgasm. Experiment with different positions as much as you like as part of "foreplay"—she'll enjoy it—but when you're serious about giving your woman an orgasm, don't expect any more of her than lying back and luxuriating in what you're doing to her.

TOO GOOD TO GO AT ANY TIME

Take your time. Start wherever you like and suck, kiss, nibble, apply hard pressure, apply short pressure, or blow (but never into the vagina, as there's a million to one chance you could give her an embolism). Work toward the clitoris, work around the sides of it, but don't touch it until her hips are writhing toward you and she's practically grabbing your ears for direction. Use a big wide lick, like you were eating ice cream. Get a lot of lubrication down there and many women will enjoy lapping more than more direct pointy-tongue action.

Remember that for lots of women the clitoris is too sensitive to take too much direct action, and that's why the big lick works so well.

How was
it for
you?

**Q   My wife never seems enthusiastic about cunnilingus. How can I
persuade her?**

A   *Usually I'd say not to push something that your wife doesn't seem to like,
but oral sex is tied up with so many body issues and shame thoughts that
lots of women just can't lie back and enjoy it—they need to be trained to
believe that it's really OK. If you seem reluctant to go down on your wife,
she may be less than interested. Having a man get up close and personal
makes women feel very vulnerable. And quite right, too. If a woman is tense
and anxious, there's absolutely no chance of her coming, so why would she
(or you) bother? She may be worrying that she'll take a long time to come.
Reassure her that you don't care. If she comes, terrific. If she doesn't, no
big deal. If I were you I wouldn't keep going for ages, not because you're a
selfish lover, but because she won't feel the performance pressure to come
if you make it clear it's part of your foreplay. Go down on her often so she
gets the idea that you like it and there's no pressure on her. With time, she
might relax enough to start enjoying it.*

Q   I don't like going down. Why should I?

A   *Well, if your partner's enjoying terrific orgasms and doesn't care, fine. But
this really is a treat for most women and to deprive your partner of it is a
shame. I take it for granted that there are no issues of hygiene here that
should be addressed first. Remember that a significant number of women can
only come this way and that the sensation is unique—when a tongue makes
you come, you know it. Women feel so happy with the person who gave them
an orgasm through oral sex that it's well worth persevering from your point of
view, too. You'll gain loads of Brownie points.*

28

Shortcuts to better orgasms

We're coming across all PC.

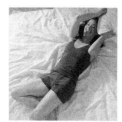

Orgasm depends on the rhythmic contraction of muscles. Train these muscles and you're going to have better orgasms.

If you're a woman, especially one who's had children, you'll be tired of discussions about your pubococcygeal (PC) muscles. These are the muscles that take a lot of the strain when you're pregnant and in labor, and so midwives and doctors stress the importance of exercising them every chance you get because without your PC muscles, to put it bluntly, you'll need diapers for longer than the baby. Hats off to Dr. Arnold Kegel, the man who first recommended these exercises to help bladder control following childbirth. But I can't help thinking that if doctors were to stress how much doing Kegels can improve your love life (for both sexes), then a lot more of us would be doing them.

Tensing and releasing these muscles increases blood flow to the genitals—and when you focus benign interest on your genitals, it tends to improve your sex life. But there's more. These are the muscles that contract during orgasm. The stronger they are, the better the contraction and the more pleasure you feel.

Here's an idea for you...

Need motivation to do your Kegels? You should notice improvements within two weeks. And within six weeks, you should feel the difference in your love life. So get clenching.

For men, strengthening your PC muscles may help you experience multiple orgasms. By having strong PC muscles you can stop on the brink of ejaculating and experience orgasm without actually coming, so you can continue to make love for longer. Exercising your PC muscles will give you better orgasms, and this is *a good thing* for men whose orgasm often seems to be less encompassing than their partner's orgasm.

FINDING YOUR PC MUSCLES

Next time you pee, stop the stream of urine mid-flow. The muscles that you're using to do that are the PC muscles. Make sure that you isolate them from the muscles surrounding the anus.

YOUR EXERCISE PROGRAM

Simply contract your PC muscles every time you remember—ten times for a couple of seconds each time. Don't overdo it and don't squeeze too hard. Aim for a steady, relaxed contraction.

Once you've got the hang of that, move up to contracting twelve times at normal speed and twelve times at a faster speed. Do this twice a day—more if you remember—for the rest of your life. And if you're really dedicated, aim for 100 Kegels a day.

FOR ADVANCED EXERCISERS

On top of your standard Kegels, try these:

■ **The elevator.** Imagine that your vagina has an elevator inside it and you're going to elevate it using your PC muscles. Take the elevator to the first floor, pause, second floor, pause, third floor, pause, top floor, pause. Now let the elevator down again. Practice and practice this, going as fast as possible and then as slowly as possible.

■ **Pelvic tilts.** Combine your Kegels with pelvic tilts, which strengthen your back and pelvis muscles so you can thrust better and for longer. Lie on the floor with your knees bent and feet flat on the floor. Contract your stomach and tilt your pelvis up, keeping your spine on the floor. Contract your PCs as you do this, hold for a couple of seconds, and then return to the beginning position. Do up to twenty tilts day.

During sex, combine Kegel action with techniques in IDEA 29, *Easy routes to faster orgasms for her.*

Try another idea...

"It is easier to keep half a dozen lovers guessing than to keep one lover after he has stopped guessing."
HELEN ROWLAND, journalist

Defining idea...

How was it for you?

Q These exercises aren't enough. Since my kids, I can barely feel a twitch when I contract my PCs. What else can I do?

A Your orgasms probably feel much weaker, too. But you can get the strength back. It's probably worth making it more of a project and setting aside a particular time each day to do your Kegels. Remember that it's not just your sex life that will benefit. After menopause, when hormonal changes make your PC muscles even weaker, you'll be grateful you took action now. You'll find it easier with something to hold on to when doing the above exercises, such as a finger, dildo, or carrot. Or you could be a little more scientific and invest in some weighted barbells—you can buy these at sex shops and over the Internet. You'll then get an indication of how weak your muscles are now and you'll be able to measure your progress as you improve. And you will.

Q So exactly how do strong PCs stop me from ejaculating?

A When you feel your PCs are strengthened, while you're masturbating try to contract them at the point just before orgasm. This stops you from ejaculating, but you should still feel pleasure. The point is you should be able to get going again after a short break. When you read up about this, it can sound a bit like a competitive sport—lots of macho bragging about never coming, being a "master of control," etc. That kind of thing worries me. But time spent learning more about your sexual response is never wasted, plus you may want to experience a multiple orgasm—who wouldn't? But it's not necessarily going to make you a better lover. Just so you know, some Eastern traditions recommend that men only come maybe once every three times they have sex. But that once is stronger, better, and more thrilling, or so they say.

29

Easy routes to faster orgasms for her

Quicker, harder, faster? How to come more easily.

Tweaking your usual lovemaking pattern can improve your sex life with a minimal amount of effort. We could have called this chapter "How to have a simultaneous orgasm," but we've always thought that was an overrated pastime. However, if you insist...

SQUEEZING

When you orgasm, your pubococcygeal (PC) muscles in the vagina contract rapidly. Tighten your PC muscles as he withdraws, and relax them as he enters. It'll take some practice but this is a recommendation from the queen of the female orgasm, Betty Dodson, who through her workshops and books has taught thousands of women how to come, and how to come better. Squeezing will jump-start your own orgasmic contractions.

Here's an idea for you... To increase your chances of simultaneous orgasm, let your partner know how excited you are and encourage the same feedback from him. If you want to minimize prosaic chat, whisper a number to your mate to let him know exactly where on a scale of 1 to 10 you are in terms of getting off. He can do the same.

PRESSING

Downward pressure on your pubic area before orgasm can increase the intensity of stimulation. Experiment with pressing down with your hand on your stomach just above your pubic bone while masturbating or using a vibrator. Then try this during intercourse. Another technique is to "bear down." This is pushing out with your PC muscles, which may help force your G-spot closer to your vaginal opening so it's likelier to get indirect stimulation from his penis.

STRETCHING

Stretching your legs flat on the bed and bringing them together while in the missionary position will increase clitoral stimulation. It works even better when you're on top. Slide your thighs down so they are over his thighs rather than his hips. Arch your back so you're bending backward. Forming an arc means you'll be putting maximum pressure on the clitoral area. Just be careful you don't bend his penis back too far—you have all the control here and, being a gentleman, he might not want to interrupt your obvious pleasure to tell you that you're in imminent danger of breaking it off.

It's also worth experimenting with other positions where you are on top and your feet are stretched down toward his feet. These tend to increase clitoral stimulation.

HANGING

Hang your head over the edge of the bed when you're having sex. The rush of blood to the brain increases sensations.

Check out the CAT position in IDEA 5, *Join the 30 percent*. It encourages clitoral stimulation.

Try another idea...

"Failing to give each other some basic direction can leave couples guessing—and frustrated. Not a big talker in bed? These four words should get you by just fine: 'faster,' 'slower,' 'harder,' and 'softer.'"
JUDY DUTTON, writing in *She* magazine

Defining idea...

How was it for you?

Q   How can we attain synchronicity? Whatever we do, I take forever to come. Unless he gets me off first, he always comes first.

A   *Hey, don't knock it! Try a vibrator. It's the easiest way to synchronize orgasms. But if you aren't happy with this or want to change it up, you could try some mind tricks. The first is to free yourself of performance pressure—fixating on having an orgasm is the surest way to stop yourself from having one. The minute the thought "God, it's taking forever" enters your mind, immediately switch off and begin to live in the moment. Come back to your body, concentrate on the sensations, and focus on your pleasure.*

Q   Why does it take women so much longer?

A   *It doesn't. It's been estimated that through intercourse it takes men eleven minutes to come and women twenty-eight minutes. (How do they know this stuff?) But let's get one thing straight. When it comes to masturbation, women come as quickly as men. So why do women take longer to come during intercourse? My theory is that men are more revved up mentally beforehand than women. A woman's orgasm will happen more quickly if you feel sexier before the action begins. After folding the ironing, don't expect to be howling orgasmically five minutes later. While your guy is still watching the news, start warming yourself up. Create your own twenty-minute ritual for separating your working day from your time with your partner. Take a shower or bath with sweet-smelling products, light candles, wear sensuous lingerie, or read a sexy story. This can make an immense difference to how quickly you orgasm.*

30

Assume the position...

...but make some changes.

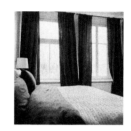

We promised no line drawings of bearded hippies doing the sort of things that bearded hippies love to do. And we're going to keep our promise.

Books of positions have always struck me as appealing predominantly to those among us who want a definitive list of every position ever known and a nice sharp pencil with which to check them off. What is generally not known is that the *Kama Sutra* was written with the elite of (male) Indian society in mind, who had nothing else to do all day but think of ways of pleasuring their personal harem. Working your way through the *Kama Sutra* ain't going to cut it with your average dual-income, too-busy-to-breathe couple. As we non-elite know, it's going to take more than a swift bout of "bending the rushes" to keep our love life exciting.

There are basically only four or five positions (no, I can't be bothered to count them), and everything else is just a variation on a theme. However, most couples find one or two favorites and stick with these because they deliver. Some simple

Here's an idea for you... **The simplest but very effective modification of the missionary position is an ancient Eastern technique: She stuffs a couple of pillows under her hips to raise her pelvis, which improves clitoral stimulation.**

modifications can make these even better. Here is a summary and some more ideas on improving on a good thing.

THREE WAYS TO MAKE A GOOD THING BETTER

Improve...the missionary

A great position, much maligned. There are two potential problems:

1. Most women won't come this way, even if he pumps away for three hours. Not unless some clitoral stimulation is brought into play.

2. He has to work harder—a lot harder.

So here's an alternative for when you both want to be on the bottom. She lies with her left leg flat on the bed and the right one bent at the knee and can lean on her elbows or prop herself up with cushions. He lies at right angles to her on his left side, supporting himself on his left arm while his lower (left leg) passes under her left thigh so he lifts up her pelvis enough to enter. She hooks her right leg over his rib cage. This should form a sort of open-scissors arrangement, which allows free access for both parties to her clitoris and means you can both gaze soulfully into each other's eyes even if you're too far away for a kiss. Movement is limited, but this is a good position for when you're feeling lazy—great for when you both have a hangover.

Improve...Her on top

Very popular position with women. Very popular with men, for that matter. Here's something to try:

She squats on top of him, then gently swivels around so that she's facing his feet. She may have to bend forward a bit and use his ankles or calves to hold on. He gets a superlative view of her bottom as opposed to her breasts. Also, if she lifts herself up between thrusts, he gets a great view of his penis entering her—probably the closest view you can get of penetration, short of a porn movie. Perhaps that's the reason this position was voted the one most men would like to try in a *Cosmopolitan* survey. And if she wriggles around, she'll get good stimulation of the area around her G-spot. Plus, few positions will give her so much scope to fantasize.

Improve...The 69

Great fun in theory, but as orgasm approaches it gets harder to concentrate on giving pleasure. One partner loses concentration, and bang, the show's over for the other one, which is one reason why couples tend to stop doing 69s once their honeymoon period is over. Remember, it's easier if you lie on your side leaning on the inside of your lover's thigh for support. You can also pass a vibrator between you so that if one of you is approaching orgasm, he or she can stop tongue action and stimulate with the vibrator instead, so that your lover stays revved up while getting you off.

I could be being a little dismissive of the power of changing positions—a book stuffed full of exotic ways to do it combined with IDEA 17, *Learn the art of kaizen*, could work well for you.

Try another idea...

"I once had a rose named after me and I was very flattered. But I was not pleased to read the description in the catalog: no good in a bed, but fine up against a wall."
ELEANOR ROOSEVELT

Defining idea...

131

How was it for you?

Q **I like standing positions, but since my husband hurt his back, I've been scared to do it. Any ideas?**

A *You could wear a pair of really high heels and lean against a wall. He'll barely have to move. They look great, too. (If you brace your hands against the wall for support, the position is sometimes called the "strip search" for obvious reasons—I'll leave it to your imagination to work out how role-play could be brought into play here.) Rear entry in general is helpful for standing positions. The easiest way is for you to bend forward and support yourself on the floor or a low table or chair. You have to be pretty supple and, for whatever reason, this is easier to accomplish in the bath with you using the sides of the tub for support. Just be careful not to slip or you'll have more than your back to worry about.*

Q **In some positions, I feel pain when my partner enters me. Why is this?**

A *He could be hitting against your cervix. General rule: The nearer your feet are to your ears, the deeper the penetration. Rear-entry positions also usually allow deep penetration (which is why they're favored by our less well-endowed brothers). By lowering your thighs during missionary-type positions, you'll be able to control the depth of his thrusting. Similarly, if you like doing rear entry, try spoon positions where you both lie side to side with him behind you—again, you'll be controlling the level of thrust. It goes without saying that if pain during sex continues it should be reported to your doctor.*

31

Betty and Daisy rather than Sadie and Missy

Or for those of you who prefer acronyms—soft-core B&D (bondage and discipline) rather than hard-core S&M (sadism and masochism).

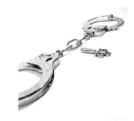

If your average Saturday night involves being spanked on a stage in front of strangers, skip over this, as I'm not going to bring anything new to your party. This chapter is aimed at people who've never really tried B&D.

WHAT'S THE POINT?

What I love about hard-core health spas—the ones where you get timetables and set menus involving lots of lentils—is that you don't have to think. You just do what you're told. That's what the submissive partner gets in B&D games. In forgoing all control, there's a whole heap of freedom.

Here's an idea for you...

For those of you who still aren't convinced about the whole B&D thing, check out a trilogy of fantasy books by Jaqueline Carey—*Kushiel's Dart* and its sequels. They're not top shelf in any way, but the heroine is a very unsubmissive masochist and the books are erotic without being porno. They might make you more eager to experiment and give you some ideas.

As for the dominant partner—what's not to love? They get to do exactly what they want, exactly the way they like it. Perfect for compulsives, who most of the time can't get the rest of us to do it their way. On our knees, on our back, tied up, tied down, or licking the heel of your shoes for twenty minutes. It's your call.

The pain you experience in these sorts of games isn't pain like when you catch your finger in the door. When pain is anticipated, it raises your heart rate and releases the feel-good hormones endorphins—just what happens during exercise. One effect of this is that you can experience heightened sexual pleasure and sensation. When things get painful, try deep steady breathing, which makes sexual sensations even stronger.

It goes without saying that all of this goes down well with a little role-play. Modify some of the scenarios in this book or make up your own. It's your night to shine. Or to be hog-tied and locked in a closet, if that's what lights your candle.

When playing with power games that involve humiliation and control there's always the chance you'll hurt another person, and I don't mean just physically. You should both agree on a word beforehand that immediately signals "game's over, time for lots of cuddling and reassurance." That word shouldn't be "no," as then you wouldn't be able to scream "please stop, oh no, you bastard," thus losing out on half the fun. It's an absolute rule that if either of you utter "the word," then you stop.

POWER GAMES

Trouble bringing this up? Turn to IDEA 16, *Think kink*, for guidance.

Try another idea...

1. **Tying up.** Play with exposure (generally, the wider the limbs are spread, the more you feel like you're open to the public—some people like that). Restraints on all four limbs are great for people who find it hard to come because of performance pressure to "get there." Restraint puts you totally at the mercy of your partner. You are in their power. They have responsibility. You can relax. Whoosh. Was that an orgasm?

2. **Spanking.** Always warm up the spankee's buttocks beforehand with some gentle slaps and then build up in a rhythmic way with gaps between strokes. The back of a hairbrush or a table tennis paddle make good alternatives if your hand is getting sore. As a general rule, never hit any part of the body that is hard. In fact, don't hit anything but the buttocks unless you know what you're doing. After administering a whupping and when the skin is still pink and tingly, run your fingers gently over their skin. This will feel exquisite.

3. **Gags.** This is more a mind thing than anything else. It looks great and it makes you feel really helpless—lots of opportunity to flail your head from side to side in best teen-slasher movie style. Tongue over the gag, please. Blindfolds work, too. The more senses you cut off—sight, speech, hearing—the more you're forced to concentrate on what you're feeling.

"The golden rule of kink: only play with people who play nice. Cause the ex who caught you cheating and now has you cuffed and blindfolded ain't comin' back."
EM and LO, sex columnists writing in *The Big Bang*

Defining idea...

135

4. **Nipple clamps.** Experiment first with nipping close to orgasm to see if it's your or your partner's thing. Those who like this really like it.

I'm assuming that when we're not dressing up as naughty schoolgirls and irate headmasters we're all sensible adults and don't need it spelled out that this is potentially dangerous stuff. No tying up for more than half an hour unless you're an expert Boy Scout. Never leave a tied up person alone without checking on them. No whips near the eyes. Enough already, I hear you say, but I know people who have done scary B&D/S&M stuff with someone who, outside of the torture chamber, they wouldn't trust to make them a sandwich. If that's you, get a grip.

Q **My husband wants me to pee on him, but I think that's disgusting. I just can't do it. Why should I?**

How was it for you?

A *Then don't. But first, and this applies to everything requested in a loving relationship, ask yourself what's going on here. Why does he want it? Why does it disgust you? By exploring, you'll find out a lot about the dynamic of the relationship. Would he settle for a simulacrum? Dr. Pam Spurr recommends some role-play before pouring body-temperature tea over your husband while he's blindfolded. Do your best, but ultimately it isn't worth it if it's going to permanently affect how you relate to your husband.*

Q **We'd like to experiment with pain, but neither of us feels comfortable with spanking. What do you suggest?**

A *There's a really bad sex scene where candles are used, starring Madonna and Willem Dafoe in a movie that's best forgotten—it's probably responsible for turning more people off than turning them on. But dripping a drop of hot wax on bare skin, then another, inflicts the right kind of pain, and it feels more grown-up than spanking. Use plain white candles (not perfumed or colored) that have just been lit (both measures ensure the wax doesn't get too hot). Hold them several feet above the skin, don't drip on the same spot repeatedly, and every now and then test yourself on your own skin to make sure the wax isn't getting too hot.*

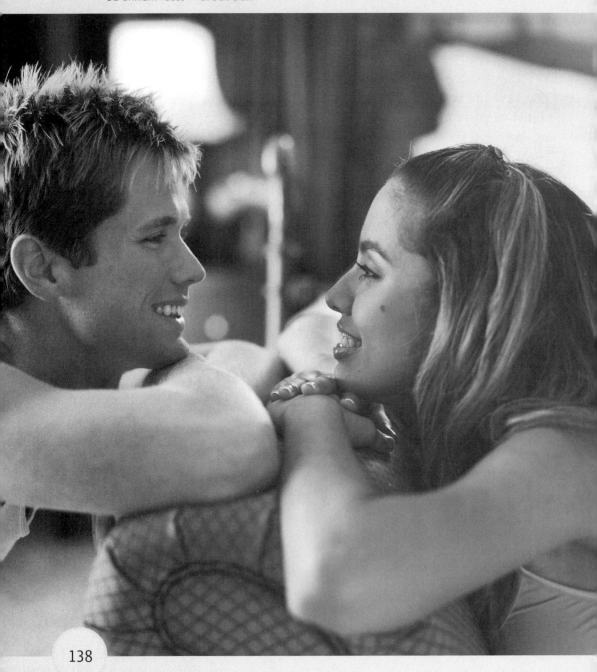

32

Heading even farther south

Few things in life will earn you so much gratitude for a moderate amount of effort.

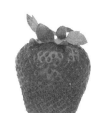

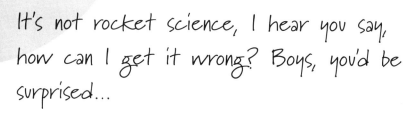

It's not rocket science, I hear you say, how can I get it wrong? Boys, you'd be surprised...

I once interviewed a woman who said she'd never enjoyed oral sex because of the biting. Biting? I queried. "Yes. He sucks so hard that his teeth get in the way." Her partner mimicked the actions of a blow job on her and it didn't occur to either of them that perhaps sucking wasn't a prerequisite. She didn't feel she could tell him he was getting it wrong so she just avoided oral sex. Nobody's suggesting that you are such a klutz, but experimentation with feedback is essential.

- First, get your partner revved up with lots of subtle kissing, licking, and teasing. This isn't just sexy, it's damn well essential. The clitoris is exquisitely sensitive. This cannot be emphasized enough. It can't take direct stimulation unless its owner is aroused. I don't suggest any man even think of approaching the clitoris (unless specifically invited) until she's thrusting her hips toward you in a pose that tells you quite explicitly what she wants.

Here's an idea for you... **Brush your hand gently through the pubic hair before getting down to business. This grooms out loose pubic hairs—less chance of them ending up between your teeth.**

- Even then, approach slowly. Most of the clitoris, the so-called clitoral arms, lie under the skin. Think of the clitoris as an inverted V, with the join being the point where you can see the clitoris. Lying along each labia, pointing downward toward the perineum, are the "arms." Think of a wishbone and stimulate all of it through the skin. The clitoris has more nerves than any other part of the body—thousands more than the penis. Direct attention can frighten it off altogether. Build up to it slowly by working on the arms of the clitoris and always check for a reaction. If she's moving her pelvis away from you, you're going at it too hard.

Defining idea... **"Some men know that a light touch of the tongue, running from a woman's toes to her ears, lingering in the softest way possible in various places in between, given often and sincerely enough, would add immeasurably to world peace."**
MARIANNE WILLIAMSON, spiritual writer and lecturer

- Try specific moves and ask your lover what variations she likes. Faster, slower, harder, softer? Side to side? Circles?

- Ask questions. Will you show me where...? Do you prefer my tongue hard or soft there? If I keep going just like this, do you think you would come? If not, do you want me to keep going anyway (hey, it's the journey not the destination)?

The secret to giving great oral sex is to remember that the recipient has to be able to concentrate. She has to stay connected to what's happening to her sexually, but still be

Turn to IDEA 27, *Heading south*, for more on cunnilingus.

Try another idea...

able to give over control entirely to you. Help her. Make sure she's comfortable. Once she's approaching orgasm, don't distract her by changing what you're doing if you're clearly doing something right.

EIGHT THINGS TO DO WITH YOUR TONGUE THAT (SOME) CLITORISES LIKE

This isn't an exhaustive list, but it's based on a poll of women asked for their favorite moves.

- Big flat licks using the whole tongue. The wetter the better.

- Flicking up the edges of the labia, eventually centering on the clitoris.

- Licking upward repeatedly along the furrows from the vagina to the clitoris, gradually pressing harder every time but never quite reaching the clitoris (stimulating the "arms," you see).

- Licking gently while pressing down just above the mons (the fleshy part directly above your nose) with the fingers.

- Circle, circle, flick, flick, flick. Circle, circle, flick, flick, flick.

- Very lazy circles around the clitoris, but not touching it. See how slow you can go. Doing this after some buildup can drive her mad with longing.

- Suck the clitoris very gently and flick your tongue over it. Or move your tongue slowly up-down, up-down.

- Make your tongue pointy and insert it into the hole rhythmically. (Author's note: This woman liked it, but many men overdo this. Remember, the clitoris is the seat of sex pleasure. Don't overdo tongue penetration unless specifically asked— assuming that their tongue should mimic their penis is the biggest technical mistake men make.)

Try all of these. And at the end when she's approaching orgasm, you'll probably be doing some version of lapping at her clitoris up and down, firmly and rhythmically in a steady and purposeful manner. She'll be bucking against you now. She might like you to hold on to her buttocks or hands tight as she approaches orgasm. It helps her concentrate. Don't change what you're doing at all except perhaps to go a little faster.

Q **He's willing, but he prods at me. Prod, prod, prod. It doesn't do anything for me. What can I tell him?**

A *First, I'd suggest that you ask him to go slowly. Really slowly. Slow and steady will eventually work for most women. (Men, if only they knew, don't usually have to go fast until the very end, and even then not always.) The point is that it's hard for him to prod slowly. It's a kind of contradiction in terms and he might automatically then start using the flat-tongue action that's more likely to work for you.*

Q **She just tells me everything's "fine." How can I get some feedback?**

A *Blindfold your lover while you're experimenting with different techniques and strokes. Often being blindfolded makes us less self-conscious in reporting how it feels. Try asking her to give each technique a mark out of ten until she gets more confident about saying what she wants or likes.*

How was it for you?

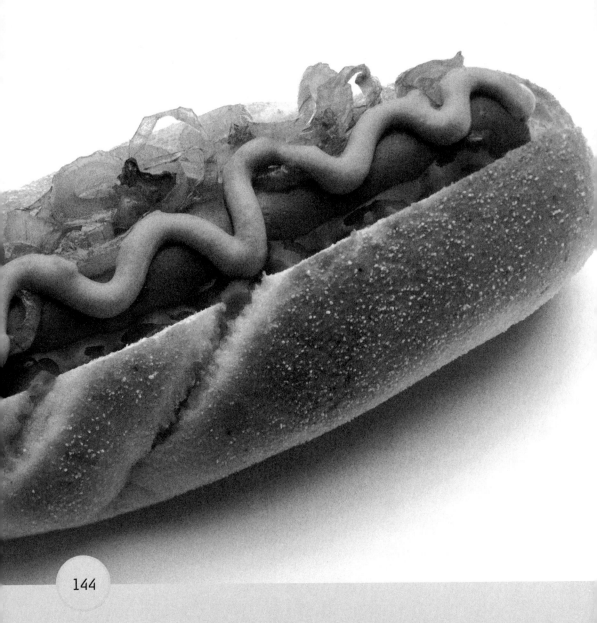

33

More on blow jobs

Can you ever know too much?

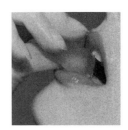

Your blow job technique comes down to just two things: what you do with your tongue, and what you do with the rest of your body.

What you can do with your tongue is limited, and most of us master the different variations—long, slow licks, flicking action, focused pressure on hot spots, etc.—pretty early on.

The magic lies in what you can do with the rest of your body while you're licking and generally pleasuring him with your mouth. Incorporate the principles of kaizen (small changes causing big differences) into your blow job technique. It's during oral sex more than just about anything else that we tend to stick to the same pattern over and over again. For a good reason—it works for our partner so why throw away a winning formula? But try mixing it up just a little and you can take a pleasurable experience into the realms of a mind-blowing experience.

Here's an idea for you... **Try stimulating the prostate gland. Men can experiment with this during masturbation and women can use it to give their man a deeper, stronger orgasm.**

HANDS

- Touch his chest; squeeze his nipples.

- Put the fingers of one hand in his mouth so he can suck and lick them.

- Trace around his anus, balls, and perineum (the space between the first two) with your fingers.

- Slip a well-lubricated finger into his butt and stimulate the prostate gland, which you can feel through the skin of the anterior wall (front), with gentle pressure (give him plenty of warning first that this is your intention). If he doesn't like this, press rhythmically on the perineum, which stimulates the prostate more gently.

- Hold tight onto his buttocks and spread the cheeks—many men, like women, appreciate the sense of stretch.

Defining idea... *"When authorities warn of the sinfulness of sex, there is an important lesson to be learned: Do not have sex with the authorities."*
MATT GROENING, creator of *The Simpsons*

- Push up the fleshy area just above the pubic bone or press on it rhythmically. This increases the sensations you're causing with your mouth.

- Put one hand on the base and another halfway up the penis. Stroke the penis with both hands while you take the head of the penis in your mouth.

- Use a vibrator or a bullet on low speed on his perineum while you fellate him.

EYES

It's oh so simple, but if you don't usually look into your lover's eyes when you go down on him, try it. A locked gaze while your mouth slides up and down is powerfully erotic. This is easier in some positions than others so alternate with holding his penis with your hand while you hold his gaze and flick your tongue over the head of his penis.

LEGS

Straddle his chest as an alternative to the usual blow job positions and go on all fours if necessary. This leaves you exposed, but visually it's pretty damn exciting, especially if you touch yourself while going south. It also allows him to touch you without any effort whatsoever, which is nice for him. On no account, however, allow him to balance his beer on your butt.

RHYTHM

Ultimately you find a technique he likes, a groove that he likes, and you stick to it. At the most, alternate between two techniques. The only exception to this is when you want to prolong things, which can ensure a stronger, better orgasm for him. Not always, however. Some men's penises appear to get bored with a constant stop–start stop–start method, and their orgasm isn't half as explosive as sex manuals would lead you to believe, so unless you know your man, don't overdo the teasing.

As someone once said, "It's not called a job for nothing." Turn to IDEA 26, *Handy work*, on hand-job techniques so you can take a break but keep stimulation seamless. Make sure you have plenty of lubricant close by.

Try another idea...

147

**Q I tried leaning my head over the edge of the bed while giving him
a blow job because I read this was the best way of deep throating.
Why didn't it work for me?**

A   *Deep throating doesn't exist, some will tell you. It certainly doesn't exist in
the '70s film starring Linda Lovelace: No woman has a clitoris on the back
of the throat. But in the sense that it means taking the whole length of a
man's penis into your mouth, then it's possible and there isn't, in fact, any
big mystique to it. It's a matter of controlling your gag reflex and this might
take some practice. The position you tried is based on porn—it's not a great
way to start because although it gives a straight line, it's no good if you
don't have the hang of overcoming the gag reflex. And, let's face it, lying
on your back while being slowly asphyxiated, with no control over the
thrusting, is likely to make you feel panicky.*

Q   So how do you deep throat?

A   *You should be in control of the penis, with your hand on the base so that
you can be quite sure of this. Keep working up and down, taking the penis
into your mouth a little at a time. When the penis hits the back of your
throat, the secret is to get the hang of the breathing. Breathe in as the
penis leaves the back of your throat, out when it hits the back of your
throat. Go a little farther every time. Once you are an expert at taking his
entire length into your mouth, you can retry with the head-hanging-off-the-
bed position, but your lover, who will be controlling the movement, is still
going to have to go gently. And never, ever believe what you see in porn or
base your performance on it.*

34

The love bath

If you're wise, the bathroom is the place to go to get dirty. Nowhere else in your house will make you feel so spa-cial. (Sorry.)

Your bathroom should be where the seduction process begins. It's the place to clean up so that you can get down—essential if you don't want to be worrying about little things like being physically repulsive to your mate.

But here's how to really make the most of your bathroom.

STEP 1: CUT LOOSE

If you find it hard to switch off and are one of those people who always has something else to do, step away from that TV or glass of wine as your evening de-stressor and instead design your own "transition ritual" where you put aside the stresses of the day and start revving up for a night of passion. It's a lot more likely to get you in the mood for sex than two hours of repeats.

Here's an idea for you... **A good bathroom pastime for women is to position your clitoris under the tap with your legs up against the wall. This can result in a powerful orgasm, but it only works if you have a mixer tap and a steady stream of hot water, of course.**

Transition rituals are especially important if you work from home (including looking after small children). Taking twenty minutes in the bathroom each night is the way you send a message to your body that the working day is over and it's time to relax, wind down, and play. Your bathroom should be as aesthetically pleasing as possible. Banish plastic toys, keep the lighting soft, and wire the bathroom for sound. Indulge in oils and lotions that make you feel good and let the cares of the day slip away as you bathe. The earlier in the evening you do this, the better. Have "transitional clothing," too: comfy, light, and sensual clothes that you feel comfortable lounging around in. Make this time for yourself—it's a lot more useful than a quick shower last thing at night or first thing in the morning.

STEP 2: HAVE SEX

If you're always too tired for sex, don't wait until it's time to sleep. You know it makes sense. Spending a little time feeling sensual by yourself when you can still keep your eyes open is going to juice you up and leave you feeling frisky. Get your partner to switch off the TV and do something equally life affirming and you'll both be in the mood. Still not convinced? OK, time for...

STEP 3: MAKE LOVE TO YOUR SHOWER

Oh all right, if you're going to be pedantic, let your shower make love to you. Seriously. If you haven't yet come with the help of your showerhead, what the hell are you doing in there? For women, especially those who have trouble orgasming, directing the flow of water from the showerhead around and on their clitoris while they're sitting on the side of the bath or lying down results in an easy orgasm. Perhaps because performance pressure is nonexistent—you don't have to worry about hurting the showerhead's feelings or taking too long—it works like a charm. When I wrote a piece about the joys of showering back in the early '90s, I was inundated with thank-you letters from women (and a few from their men) who had read the piece and headed straight for the local hardware store, with fabulous results. So, if you're looking for a good reason to install a decent shower, make it your love life.

Men can enjoy teasing with a showerhead, too—slowly increase the pressure to a point that feels fantastic.

Note that women should only point the showerhead downward. Water forced up into the vagina carries a very, very small risk of forcing an air bubble where you really don't want one. Not good.

The bathroom can be a good place to put IDEA 46, *Wait. We said wait!*, into practice. You can move the action to the bedroom to really prolong things.

Try another idea...

"Why are women wearing perfumes that smell like flowers? Men don't like flowers. I've been wearing a great new scent guaranteed to attract men. It's called New Car Interior."
RITA RUDNER, comedian

Defining idea...

How was it for you?

Q   **I tried this lying in the bath underwater and came—eventually. But it takes a long time. How can I speed things up?**

A   *It may take you longer than other methods. That's part of the charm. If you're in a hurry, try one of the vibrators that are water-resistant.*

Q   **We like the transitional ritual idea. Any more ideas?**

A   *It works even better as a de-stressor if you do it together. You could pamper each other in the bathroom. Try rubbing each other down with gritty exfoliators or smoothing oils over each other's bodies. Aim for multiple sensory experiences and generally give each other a bit of TLC before hopping into the shower and having sex. As I keep saying, this is terrific for couples who are always too tired at 11 p.m. For special occasions, put some old towels on the bathroom floor and get really mucky. Dribble honey, chocolate sauce, cream, or Bailey's all over each other and lick it off. And when that gets boring, there's your old friend the showerhead itching to join the party.*

35

Fight club

Sexual energy isn't the only flow of energy between a long-standing couple. There's blind fury, too.

Some couples need a fight to lift their energy enough to have sex, some find their best sex is after a fight, and some like "make-up" sex so much that they pick fights to get turned on.

This last one isn't recommended as it can be emotionally wearing, but you can still use a fight to your best advantage.

WHEN A FIGHT IS NOT A FIGHT

A fight is not just a fight when it's a way of raising your energy and sparking excitement between the pair of you.

- When you're tired, do you find just having your partner in the room deeply irritating?

Here's an idea for you... **Welcome fights as an opportunity to improve your relationship. A couple's ability to use disagreements to air problems and reach a compromise that brings them closer is one of the signs of a good relationship.**

■ After a period of being happy with your partner, do you feel a sort of pressure building up—a need to get some extreme reaction from them?

■ When you're bored, do you find yourself enjoying an argument about politics, the neighbors, the social significance of Ikea, whatever, as long as you can take up a diametrically opposite position from your mate?

Answer yes to any of these? If so, you may be a lover, but you're also a fighter.

■ Do you sometimes feel picked on, that no matter what you do, your partner is going to seek you out and find fault?

■ Do you have fights that blow up out of nowhere? You're looking out the window, watching the flowers grow, and suddenly you're spitting at each other?

■ Have you noticed that your partner is always particularly loving after a blowup between you?

Yes? You've got yourself a fighter.

There's no advice here on avoiding fights. A good fight, fought cleanly, can do a lot for a relationship, not least of which is giving you the chance to make up afterward. There's nothing wrong with harnessing that negative energy and converting it into passion of another type.

If your fights are fast veering from the recreational to the psychotic, read IDEA 49, *Dealing with burnout.*

Try another idea...

But the important thing is to recognize when you're having a fight purely to raise the energy because then you can maximize the fun. When a fight is brewing, decide whether it's about something important. Is one of you making a point fundamental to your relationship? Or is it simply a blowup, a release of energy, a way of letting off steam at one of the few people that it's "safe" to lose it with?

If the fight's about something important, you need to know how to fight cleanly and work toward a resolution:

- Don't generalize ("Women always do…"/"You always say…"), test ("If you loved me…"), name-call ("You're horrible"), or blame ("You made me…").

- Do stick to the present ("This time…"), stick to the first person ("I feel…" rather than "You make me…"), and look to compromise ("What do we need to both be happy?").

"Don't go to bed angry. Stay up and fight."
PHYLLIS DILLER, comedian

Defining idea...

If it's the letting off steam option—woo-hoo! You still have to fight cleanly, but you can also have some fun.

■ Keep to all the rules above.

■ When it's getting heated and you both feel the need for some time out, move the action to the bedroom.

■ The *Kama Sutra* suggests eight different ways of biting and four ritual blows before intercourse. It's very big on scratching, too. Proof, if any were needed, that getting physical isn't anything new. Gentle thumping, pushing each other around, getting rough, using your body to express your anger at your mate are all OK. Go for it, but remember it's for fun no matter how angry you are. When we're sexually excited, we have a heightened ability to handle pain—ask the spankees among us. So, be careful not to overdo it just because your partner's not screaming in pain. They simply might not be feeling it yet.

Q   **We don't fight. We just gripe at each other. How can we fight "correctly"?**

How was it for you?

A   *When you find yourself bickering a lot and generally getting on each other's nerves, forget the verbal and get physical. Retire to the bedroom and resolve problems the old-fashioned way—with pillows. Other alternatives if you have more time include:*

- ■ ***Naked wrestling.*** *Use lots of baby oil and fight on the bed. The first one to force the other off the bed wins. Make it the best of three falls.*
- ■ ***Strip wrestling.*** *First one to get the other naked wins. If you're very unequally matched physically, the larger should be handicapped with a blindfold or one-handed.*
- ■ ***Tease torture.*** *One of you is tied to a seat and has to keep a straight face while the other does all he or she can to make you smile.*

Q   **Our fights are always serious and bad-tempered. No amount of pillow fights are going to help us out. What's wrong?**

A   *If you're fighting continually, there's almost certainly an underlying resentment—either one of you is angry or both of you. Couples often put up smoke screens to distract them from facing what's really upsetting them. They'll argue about whether they can afford a new car when what they're really angry about is a lack of sex, commitment, or affection. It's a control thing—one person is holding tight to the power in the relationship. The solution? You can try being brave and saying, "We're arguing about stupid things because we can't agree about this big thing. Let's figure it out." It's the grown-up thing to do, but if your partner won't talk, all you can do is carry on with your life and as far as possible not react to their attempt to withdraw or control.*

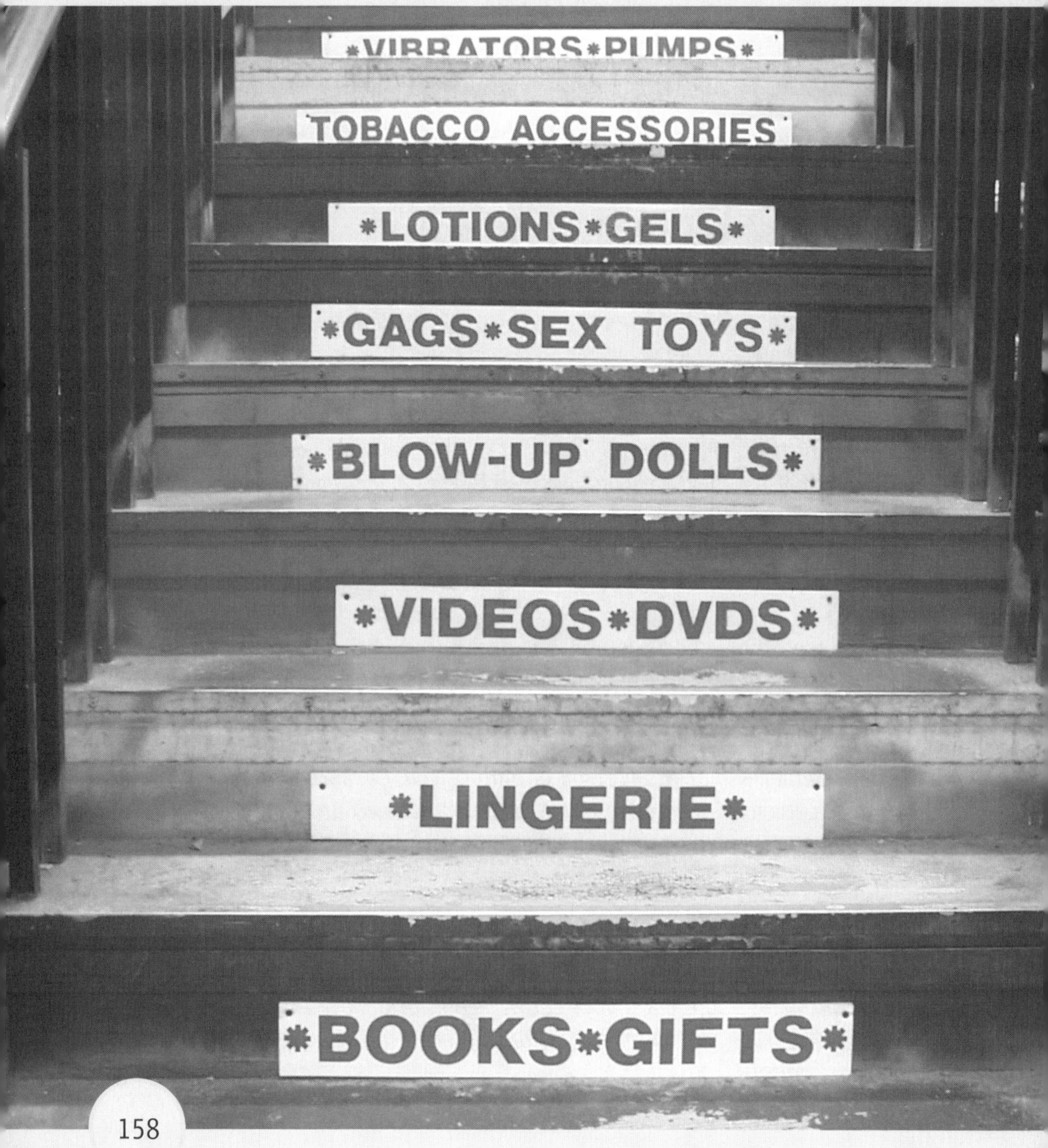
*VIBRATORS*PUMPS*
TOBACCO ACCESSORIES
*LOTIONS*GELS*
*GAGS*SEX TOYS*
BLOW-UP DOLLS
*VIDEOS*DVDS*
LINGERIE
*BOOKS*GIFTS*

36

The joy of shopping

Who knew that going to the store could be so good for your love life?

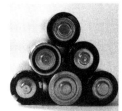

For some women, their vibrator is a good and trusty friend with whom they hang out often. For others, it's a tacky piece of plastic hidden in the nightstand drawer.

This chapter is for the latter, because clearly, although your love life may be buzzing, it's not buzzing literally, and that could mean you're missing a trick. A vibrator is a good and useful thing—a fun thing for both of you. The point of a vibrator is that, yes, it vibrates. Most usefully against your clitoris. To do that it doesn't matter what shape it is, but it helps if it fits on your finger and is pretty discreet so it doesn't get in the way, i.e., not a massive throbbing eight-inch copy of a dick. Funnily enough, what works well for you will probably work well for your guy, too. You can use it during sex to run up and down his penis or vibrate against his perineum.

Here's an idea for you...

For detailed advice on sex toys of all descriptions, access www.sh-womenstore.com; www.babeland.com and www.xandria.com also have a good selection.

Here are some vibrators worth checking out. All of these were recommended by the wonderful Kathryn, who works at Sh! (pronounced "shush"), the first UK sex shop aimed at women.

1. **Your finger—but improved!** The TantraBeam slips over your finger like a ring. It makes your finger vibrate so you can touch skin on skin. Good for people who like to keep things natural.

2. **Remote control.** Toys like the Mantric consist of a small bullet that can be held against any part of your body and a control pack that offers a whole handful of different combinations of stimulation. Or you can buy strap-on vibes that fit discreetly over her clitoris. Try spooning each other while he controls the vibration that she's feeling and, ultimately, when she comes. If he enters her for the last part, he'll feel the vibrations, too.

   Another gadget (The Octupus for him and The Oyster for her) is worn in your pants but is controlled by a remote control that your partner holds. You can give them a blast while they're wandering around the house, talking to the neighbor, having dinner in a restaurant. Not while driving the car.

3. **Rings of confidence.** Cock rings fitted around the penis keep it engorged—good for her, good for him. When the cock ring has a clitoral stimulator attached to it, things get even better. There are lots of these, but one that's definitely worth checking out is the Touchmatic, which only vibrates when it touches the clitoris.

On-off, on-off as he goes in-out, in-out. Interesting sensation, if a little distracting, but some people absolutely love it.

Turn to IDEA 37, *Play away*, for more on sex toys.

Try another idea...

4. **G-vibes.** There are a whole range of vibrators that are designed to hit your G-spot, such as the G-Swirl. This is made from silicone, which suits more people than rubber or plastic, even if it's a bit more expensive. Or there's Natural Contours Ultime.

Back in the 19th century, vibrators existed before irons and vacuum cleaners. Electric versions were invented PDQ in order to relieve exhausted doctors who were often requested to get off their female patients by hand as a medical procedure to relieve the symptoms of hysteria. I'm not making this up. Vibrators soon got popular with the public, since paying your doctor for a hand job was pretty expensive, not to say pretty embarrassing. And things have just gotten better ever since.

The sex-toy industry improves all the time. The day I visited Sh! they were excited by the imminent arrival of a new sort of vibrating condom, which their tester and her man were enthusiastic about. So, if your last venture into sex shopping was in your teens for a dare when you emerged with a totally useless red-and-black garter, do yourself a favor, as times have moved on.

Defining idea...

"Couples have to liberate masturbation, accept self-pleasuring in each other, show one another how to do it. And if a man can't handle seeing his lover use a vibrator, my advice to the woman is: Keep the vibrator and recycle the man."
BETTY DODSON, sex guru

How was it for you? **Q Is it true that you can become desensitized through using vibrators?**

A *According to Kathryn, you can. You find you can only come through a certain amount of vibration, delivered by a certain kind of vibrator, delivered in an exact way. Which is clearly a pain. The answer is—just like any other sexual partner—don't get lazy with your vibe. Try different kinds of vibrators, alter the way you masturbate, do it through a layer of clothing, take longer and use a lower setting, ask your partner to use it on you. Toys that supply different speeds and settings are good for keeping your genitals on their toes, so to speak. If you can only come with your vibrator, experiment with other ways of doing it just for the hell of it. Don't get into a rut.*

Q My last vibrator was really noisy. Do you have any recommendations?

A *Silicone vibrators are better than plastic ones. These days some are whisper quiet. Sh! gives a loudness value. But remember the point is to get off— some women need a lot of stimulation and sometimes that means a lot of revs. No namby-pamby vibrator is going to do it for the majority of us. So to hell with the noise, turn up the music!*

Play away

It's safe to say that about ten seconds after some bright cave dweller discovered that the carrot was good to eat, another one figured out that it was good for something else, too.

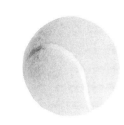

Sex toys are some of the oldest toys we've got. And they're not called toys for nothing. They're fun. Great fun. Embrace them.

Every couple should have their own "treasure chest"—a special, locked box into which they can dip for a little inspiration. What to put in it? Go shopping. It makes a great date. You might want to go virtual shopping, which is more discreet, and if you get on the Internet now you can be playing with your new toy within forty-eight hours. Here are some ideas.

LUBE

And loads of it. Kathryn from my favorite sex shop Sh! says, "Lesbians have never had the hang-up about lube that straight couples do. Using lube doesn't mean you're not a hot vixen. It makes everything better, especially if you want a good long session."

Here's an idea for you... **If you enjoy him sucking on your clitoris, you may enjoy a clit pump that can be (gently) used to plump up the tissues around the clitoris, rendering them exquisitely sensitive.**

Lush is a slightly cheaper version of the famous Liquid Silk, and Probe is a great lubricant for those with allergies. Kathryn recommends Escalate, which contains L-arginine, a natural substance that encourages blood flow and increases sexual pleasure. L-arginine is terrific, but it isn't recommended for people with herpes, as there's a small chance it may aggravate them.

If you use any latex products for contraception, don't use Vaseline, baby oil, or anything else that will eat up the rubber.

DILDOS AND STRAP-ONS

"We sell about 30–40 percent of our strap-ons (harnesses) to heterosexual couples," says Kathryn, dispelling forever the idea that it's just lesbians with a bad case of penis envy that like waving dildos around the bedroom. She continues, "It's not a fantasy role-play thing, I don't think. I reckon it's straightforward sensation. Men are getting in touch with their prostate." Ladies, look out for slip-on harnesses, like a neat Velcro G-string that gives a snugger fit than many other harnesses, so there's no flapping about.

There are so many different types of dildos, but the serious choice is silicone—expensive but feels great and heats to body temperature quickly.

And if you want the sensations but can't be bothered with the whole harness thing, look out for the Sh! version of a famous sex toy that they thought they could improve upon. Basically, it's a weighted double dildo where the woman holds one end inside her using her PC muscles, which will give her G-spot stimulation, while the other end penetrates her partner.

Turn to **IDEA 36**, *The joy of shopping*, for Internet addresses for discreet shopping.

Try another idea...

COMING FROM BEHIND

Butt plugs don't provide any motion but they give your anal muscles something to react against when you come. Comforting to wear around the house while doing chores, I'm told. If you like repeated contraction and relaxation of these same muscles then try some beads that when whipped out slowly, or all at once at the point of orgasm, give the prostate a great workout. And, of course, you can buy long, thin vibrators specially designed for anal stimulation.

"There are a number of sexual devices which increase sexual arousal, particularly in women. Chief among these is the Mercedes-Benz 380SL convertible."
P. J. O'ROURKE

Defining idea...

How was it for you?

Q Any porn that might heat up our love life?

A   *I wish.*

Q No, seriously. Isn't there *anything* you can recommend?

A   *Sorry to be so flippant, but I believe that women are just as visual as men when it comes to sex, they just lack anything good to look at. Some porn designed to turn on men also turns on women, so experiment. But many of us start to feel lousy after a while—our bodies react physically to it, but the relentless misogyny just gets us down and our minds start to switch off. You could try looking at porn aimed at lesbians, as you might find something that turns you both on. Some adult education videos are supposed to be pretty good. Or maybe you could buy the book* Erotic Home Video *by Anna Span and make your own adult films.*

38

Danger

Danger is the fastest-acting aphrodisiac.

This works better than porn—
no kidding.

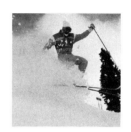

In a famous experiment, an attractive scientist interviewed two groups of men. The first group had a standard interview. The second were interviewed after they'd crossed a particularly dangerous rope bridge. By the time they were interviewed, their palms were sweaty and their hearts were beating fast. This group of men found the same interviewer significantly more alluring. The danger had heightened their sexual response.

In another experiment, male volunteers were each assigned an attractive female assistant. They were told the experiment was investigating electric shock treatments. Some men were told they were in the control group so they wouldn't be receiving shocks. The rest were told they were going to receive painful jolts of electricity. Then they were asked how attracted they felt to their research partner. The ones who were nervously awaiting the shocks found the same women significantly more attractive than the control group.

Here's an
idea for
you...

That old chestnut of making a list of six escapades to try and then letting a dice decide which you'll undergo together brings a delicious thrill of Russian roulette to the proceedings.

I couldn't find any similar experiments carried out on women, but I'm sure the results would be pretty much the same. Danger works, most probably, on two levels. First, being scared makes life seem more intense and heightens sexual desire along with everything else. Secondly, it's the old caveman thing. Share danger together and the guy gets the chance to look after the female, and she gets to feel all fragile and protected even if she's a cutthroat investment banker who fries balls before breakfast in real life.

No one's suggesting that you set yourself up for anything life threatening, but sharing adventures together will do the job—especially physical adventures. Adventures count as anything that gets your adrenaline flowing. It needn't necessarily be dangerous. You're simply seeking a shared experience that gets both of your hearts thumping.

SOME-IDEAS

Soft-core

- Go to Disneyland or anywhere with fast, high rides.
- Dare each other.
- Have sex where you might just be seen.
- Stay the night somewhere reputedly haunted, but definitely creepy.
- Shop at a sex shop together.

Hard-core

- Have sex when other people could definitely see you. (Be subtle—you don't want to frighten people or get arrested.)
- Go white-water rafting, bungee jumping, or parachute jumping.
- Take your clothes off at midnight at the end of your street.
- Go to amateur night at your local comedy club together. Stand up and be funny.

Use your imagination. Combine danger with secrecy in IDEA 42, *Dirty little secrets*, for some extremely bonding experiences.

Try another idea...

Finally, actively trying to instill a sense of danger to your lives should act as an aphrodisiac, but to strengthen the bond between you and not just the sexual energy, look at the totality of the life you're building together. If you're experiencing sexual doldrums, is that because your life has become stale and everything's routine? As a couple, are you building the sort of life you want? Is it time to stop playing at being dangerous and start taking some genuine risks with the intention of improving your life? Is it time to move to the country, move to the city, change jobs, have a child, adopt a child, travel around the world, give up work and live off the land, start a new business, live on a beach? Sure, it's frightening. Sure, it might backfire. But if you can agree on a huge life-changing, scary-as-hell decision together and you succeed, your satisfaction with each other should be sky-high. And there's nothing like feeling that you've worked hard and succeeded at something with your soul mate for giving your libido a bit of a boost.

"My ultimate fantasy is to entice a man to my bedroom, put a gun to his head, and say 'make babies or die.'"
RUBY WAX, writer and comedian

Defining idea...

Q **My partner is just not the type for this. He's an intellectual kind of guy and all your ideas are outdoorsy. What else can I try?**

A *Hmm. I see your point. Try doing things differently, possibly pushing him out of his comfort zone a little. For example, suggest that you meet at the Prada in Madrid on a particular Saturday next month. You have to get there alone. You're not allowed to confer in any way. Travel separately and check in to separate hotels. Meet. It's not exactly dangerous but you'll have each have had separate experiences, met different people, and had to think outside the box—a first step to living more exciting lives.*

Q **We have different danger levels. Going horse riding is pretty scary for me, but my boyfriend wants to go parachute jumping. Surely being terrified won't help?**

A *That's sort of the idea, but for goodness sake don't be foolhardy or you'll end up hating him. Start with horse riding. Go at your own speed. Competence builds confidence. Make sure he realizes that horse riding is just as scary for you as parachute jumping is for him.*

39

Let a woman be a woman and a man be a man

There's a man named David Deida who has some interesting ideas as to why sex goes off the rails.

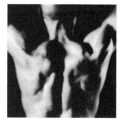

There's nothing particularly new about his ideas, but the way he packages his theories is pretty compulsive.

We're equal, but we're tired. Even long-standing relationships are crumbling under the strain of couples overworking. The latest figures show that the divorce rate is inching toward half of all marriages.

But according to Deida, life doesn't have to be this way. Deida says women aren't drudges, but passionate, vital, thrilling creatures who, given the chance, should be living a life of rich emotional complexity. In order to shine, they need the love of what Deida calls "the superior man." A strong, focused, individual striving toward his destiny. According to Deida, when men are strong and women can rely on them, passionate intensity isn't far away. What's wrecking our sex lives, he says, is too much equality. Yes, you read that right.

Here's an idea for you... **David Deida has written several books, including *The Way of the Superior Man* (for men) and *It's a Guy Thing* (for women). You can check out www.deida.com to see if his ideas appeal to you.**

"The bottom line of today's fifty–fifty relationship," Deida continues, "is that men and women are clinging to a politically correct sameness even in bed and that's when sexual attraction disappears. The love may be strong, but the sexual polarity fades." According to Deida, men and women have both a masculine and feminine side or "polarity." It's fine for men to get in touch with their feminine side (real men do cry), and women with their masculine (they're brilliant in the boardroom). She can be the breadwinner, he can look after the kids, but if they want fireworks to continue, he has to be someone she can rely on and trust, and she has to remove the shoulder pads as soon as she walks through the front door.

WHAT'S A SUPERIOR MAN?

Deida's roots appear to be in the men's movement, the reaction to feminism, which tries to help men make sense of our crazy, mixed-up world, and their role in it. He believes that a man isn't really happy unless he's striving toward his goal, whatever that is. When he loses sight of his goal, he needs "time out"—what in other cultures would have been called a "vision quest"—metaphorically speaking, going into the desert and beating his drum until he finds his way again. Unless he finds his way he's no use to anyone, least of all his lady. This is why she has to understand the importance of his quest. She can also help him be a superior man by "challenging him," i.e., not putting up with any shit. No lying about watching sports when he should be looking for a job. No nights down at the bar to distract him from the fact that he hasn't written a word of that bestselling novel. Deida calls it "challenging." It sounds like plain old "nagging" to me. Anyway, there's lots in his work about how a man can become superior, but here's a couple of ways he can be superior in direct relation to the woman in his life.

Turn to IDEA 52, *Are you sexually mature?*, to check just how evolved you are when it comes to relating to each other.

Try another idea...

You'll know you're a superior man when you stop trying to control a woman's emotions and you listen to her. You do your best to understand her feelings and don't walk away from them. You don't offer useless advice when she wants you as a sounding board, but give her a hug. You make her laugh a lot. You're your own man. You listen, you take advice on board and then you do what you think is best. You're trustworthy. You do what you say you'll do. And when you don't, you own up and take responsibility for it. You pay attention to your partner. You know that thirty minutes fully concentrating on her is worth four hours half-listening and fiddling with the remote. Got that?

Deida's ideas aren't for everyone, but I've met and interviewed couples for whom his ideas work well. The couples are equal, but they accept that the sexes are different and that a man and a woman can't be everything to each other. Deida's ideas give a way of negotiating the contradictions of being a "good guy" and being a "new man," which lots of men struggle with. If you can handle the New Age language, of course.

"Both men and women are bisexual in the psychological sense. I shall conclude that you have decided in your own minds to make 'active' coincide with 'masculine' and 'passive' with 'feminine.' But I advise against it."
SIGMUND FREUD

Defining idea...

How was it for you?

Q **Let me get this right. I have to wander around like a drippy hippie, supporting his "quest"?**

A *No, he can support your quest. Couples can switch polarity completely, and as long as that works for you, and the polarity is present, fine. But most of us switch between polarities and the danger lies where a woman is expected to carry too much of the masculine energy and can't switch back into being feminine. Who can doubt that many women these days are dazed and confused, attempting to do too much and taking out their frustration on their men? Your aspirations are important, too. But for your relationship's sake, you need to keep polarity and keep in touch with your "sense of identity."*

Q **And what would that be exactly?**

A *A woman should nourish her femininity at every opportunity—dancing, music, yoga, hanging out with girlfriends, orgasmic sex. All of these will support your feminine essence, and making time for them should be a priority if you want your relationship to stay strong. Do some nourishing every day. Have a long luxurious bath, dress in silk or other sensuous fabric, massage with scented oils, play your favorite music and dance like no one's watching, or stare at the stars. Spend as much time as possible with supportive women friends, as they can often see what you need better than you can. And before you ask, your partner has to actively help you find the time for these things. That's the superior way.*

40

Tantric sex

Not just for Sting.

If you have absolutely had it with your partner's idea of foreplay being a quick tap on your shoulder and a hopeful expression, then it's time to go Tantric.

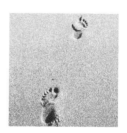

To the student of Tantra, sex is sacred, a means of accessing your spirituality and a way to meditate, transcend your problems, and reach a happier, more blissful state. For those of us who don't have the time or inclination to study Tantric sex in any great depth, it can still add a lot. It teaches sex is important, and by clearing time to undergo a few of the simpler rituals you declare to each other, "Hey, our sex life is a priority."

Tantric sex teaches you to concentrate on your lover and on the sensations that you're feeling. Forget the orgasm. The journey, not the arrival, is what's important. And for that reason alone, Tantra can be liberating and mind-altering, even if you don't get into it the whole way.

Here's an idea for you... **Try dreaming of rain forests, droning music, an overflowing bank account...once you're out of Sting-world though, Google "Tantric," but set your porn filter to "Kill."**

RITUAL 1: CREATE A "TEMPLE OF LOVE"

A really simple method of foreplay is to make your bedroom a sensual haven quite different from the rest of your home. You don't have to opt for lurid leopard prints and black walls—unless you like that, of course—but take a long look at your bedroom as if seeing it for the first time. Does is say "love," "passion," "excitement"? Is it a room devoted to the two of you?

First, think about what's in the room. Would you say that the television contributed to improving your love life? Unless you mainly use it to watch porn, probably not. Perhaps you spend more time watching it than talking to each other. If you want to keep the TV, find a scarf to cover it as a mental signal that you're switching off from the outside world. Similarly, ban work paraphernalia—piles of clothes waiting to be ironed, family photographs, anything that takes your attention away from each other and onto your responsibilities. Repair and clean ratty or old furnishings. Clear away clutter. Throw open the windows and let some fresh air circulate. This room is a reflection of your relationship—it's where you spend the most time with each other. It should sparkle.

Finally, create a love altar. Find a picture of you both together that symbolizes the best of your relationship. When you look at it, you should feel warm and compassionate toward your partner and strong as a couple. Place it in a nice frame where you can see it easily every day. Keep fresh flowers next to the photograph and candles—anything that you have to tend regularly and pay attention to—as a

physical reminder that your relationship needs
similar care and tending. Make sure there are
soft lights in your bedroom, soft music on
hand, and comfortable cushions or duvets that
you can sink into. A bedroom should always be comfortably warm so hanging
around with few clothes on doesn't make you shudder.

Turn to IDEA 41, *In out, in out,* for more Tantric-type ideas.

Try another idea...

None of this is genius level, but think of your and your friends' bedrooms. How
many have been designed with sensuality, luxury, comfort, and *sex* in mind? Your
bedroom should be a place that's welcoming to both of you, so that you look
forward to hanging out in the only place where most couples can be truly intimate
and private with each other.

RITUAL 2: THINK YOURSELF IN LOVE

Tantric sex depends on visualization to build sexual energy. As your lover begins to
caress you, feel how much they love you. Imagine their love for you flowing from
their fingers and hands and nurturing you.
Melt into their embrace. When they kiss you,
feel that with each kiss they are showing how
much they love you. Imagine the sexual energy
that you are creating between you is visible as a
red or pink light emanating from your genitals
and surrounding you like a force field of love.
As your partner touches you, imagine that your
arousal is growing like a great wave of light. See
it as fire or energy emerging from your deep

"The relation of man to a woman is the flowing of two rivers side by side, sometimes mingling, then separating again, and traveling on. The relationship is a lifelong change and lifelong traveling."
D. H. LAWRENCE

Defining idea...

177

pelvis and adding to the force field surrounding and supporting you. As you begin to have sex, imagine the energy passing upward from the base of your spine to your heart and feel this energy as love around your heart—feel it as joy—and imagine it reaching out and surrounding your partner's heart. Then, as you get more excited, imagine the energy being drawn upward and flowing out through the top of your head.

That's the way to enlightenment, but it takes some practice. Look on the bright side; with all that visualizing going on at least you won't be thinking about who's doing the school run tomorrow.

How was it for you?

Q   It feels good, but it doesn't feel that special. Why not?

A   *Tantric sex is a discipline—with practice, the feelings grow. If you believe in the basic concept that sex is a way to deepen and enrich your life, then invest in a good book about Tantric sex.*

Q   Does it mean you can last for hours?

A   *Er, yes. That's part of it. With practice, couples can keep going for hours if that's what they want. But even Sting, the most famous proponent of Tantric sex, cracked the joke that when he'd gone public about his seven-hour sex sessions, he hadn't mentioned that five and a half hours were taken up with dinner and a movie. Don't get too attached to the outcome of lasting all night. That's not the point.*

41

In out, in out

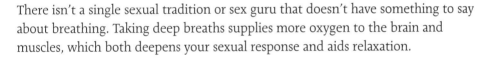

**Breathing. You do it every single minute of your life.
Boy, have you been taking it for granted!**

With the least amount of effort, you can turn the simple act of breathing into a way to heighten sexual pleasure and get closer to your partner. Pretty damn useful.

There isn't a single sexual tradition or sex guru that doesn't have something to say about breathing. Taking deep breaths supplies more oxygen to the brain and muscles, which both deepens your sexual response and aids relaxation.

FIRST THINGS FIRST

Next time you're having sex, breathe as normal and observe what you do. Olivia St. Claire, author of *302 Advanced Techniques for Driving a Man Wild in Bed*, says most women breathe shallowly when they're having sex. Taking deeper breaths should deepen sensations, but can be hard to remember when approaching orgasm. At that point, try instead to take rapid, deep breaths through your mouth rather than your nose.

Here's an idea for you... **If you're wound up, try using breathing techniques to de-stress yourself. They're the basis of all meditation, as well as improved sex.**

Men, too, can deepen sensation by breathing deeply. Both of you imagine that you are drawing air down through your lungs into your pelvic area. Concentrating your attention there via your breathing can help build excitement.

THE "COMPLETE" BREATH

Yogic breathing is to draw breath in, hold the breath in your lungs, exhale, and then pause before breathing again. Practice this and then breathe in for one count, hold for four counts, breathe out for two counts and pause. Repeat this until it comes naturally.

FOCUSING ON LOVE

In the Tantric tradition, the inward breath is associated with energy and the outward breath with consciousness. This is a good basis for a mini-meditation session before you make love. Concentrate on taking energy in with each inward breath and, with each outward breath, bringing your concentration to bear on how you're feeling right here, right now.

Defining idea... *"There is only one real antidote to the anguish engendered in humanity by its awareness of inevitable death: erotic joy."*
BENEDIKT TASCHEN, German publisher

BREATHING IN UNISON

I was once asked to write a piece about improving communication between lovers. My partner and I were given around twenty techniques to try out that were supposed to help improve our relationship. One was to lie in bed, "spooned" around each other, and simply breathe in unison. During the two weeks that we undertook our "research," we spent hours writing lists, talking deeply, having sex at odd times and in odd positions, massaging each other, and even venturing to a salsa class, but probably nothing worked as elegantly as the simple breathing exercise. Nothing else stuck either. Try it once a day (oh, all right then, as often as you remember), in bed or out, clothed or not. Hold on to each other and regulate your breaths. Let thoughts drift away as they float into your mind. Just be with each other.

For those who like this, try heart breathing. Sit on your bed in a comfortable position facing each other. Place your hands flat on your chest between your breasts (above the heart chakra). Close your eyes. Now breathe as detailed under "The 'complete' breath" above. Imagine you're drawing love in with each breath and, while holding it in your lungs, feel it nourishing your body and spirit. Finally, when you breathe out imagine your breath leaving your body as a wave of love rolling over and around your partner. Open your eyes and look at your partner while you breathe together.

If you want to make sex more spiritual, turn to IDEA 40, *Tantric sex.*

Try another idea…

Defining idea…

"Your breath is a bridge between your body, feelings and thoughts, your energy, your past and your present. How we breathe directly affects every cell of our body, and it also influences how we feel emotionally. As such, the breath is also a vehicle for expansion and ecstasy."
LEONORA LIGHTWOMAN, Tantric teacher and author

How was it for you?

Q **Very relaxing, but how does this relate to improving sex?**

A *The more relaxed or "open" that you are, the more likely you are to be in touch with your body. Breathing deeply and feeling yourself "expand with love," helps you feel more powerfully aware of your sexuality and anyone else's who happens to be in the room. David Deida says that deep breathing is especially important for women, and is one of the ways of maintaining their feminine polarity. He urges us as often as possible—all day, preferably—to "breathe with the same open pleasure you would if your lover's body were pressing against yours." Not easy, but work at it and Deida promises both "men and women will be attracted to your radiance and respectful of your depth." In other words, you'll be more serene and less stressed, which does indeed tend to be more attractive than the alternative—a fried wreck. But seriously, imagining you are relaxing into a loving embrace during the day, especially when things get frantic, acts to make you think of your lover, sex, hugs, and physical closeness—all the good things in life. And yes, it boosts your libido.*

Q **I start to get giddy after a while. Is this OK?**

A *This proves you're doing it right. These exercises or similar ones are the basis of all the mystic traditions. Because breathing is the one thing we can't forget to do, "working with the breath," basically becoming conscious of our breathing, has been used since time began as a means of making us aware that we are alive in this moment, and there won't be another one quite like it. Recalling that self-evident fact is a powerful way of appreciating life in general and your lover in particular.*

42

Dirty little secrets

Why every couple needs some.

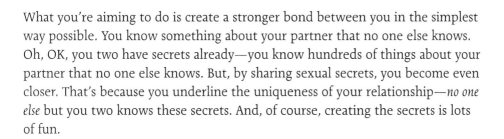

Think about the best vacation you've ever had together. Those shared memories can't help but make you smile. And no one else would understand them but you two. This chapter is about the sex equivalent of the perfect vacation.

What you're aiming to do is create a stronger bond between you in the simplest way possible. You know something about your partner that no one else knows. Oh, OK, you two have secrets already—you know hundreds of things about your partner that no one else knows. But, by sharing sexual secrets, you become even closer. That's because you underline the uniqueness of your relationship—*no one else* but you two knows these secrets. And, of course, creating the secrets is lots of fun.

Here's an idea for you... **Create new sexual secrets. Talk about old ones that you've shared. On no account share the sexual secrets you had with another partner. That's missing the point.**

A good example of creating a sexual secret is to shave off each other's pubic hair. This is still mildly shocking, though God knows why with the ubiquity of the Brazilian wax, where both sexes let total strangers loose on them. Whatever. Besides the thrill of naughtiness, there's a practical reason to try shaving. Being hairless increases sensations, especially during oral sex. Plus, in a crowded room, you'll be the only one who knows why your partner is squirming about so much in his or her seat when the hair starts to regrow. But despite the itch, it's well worth trying at least once because it really redefines the meaning of "intimacy." First, trim with small nail scissors (you see why this is so intimate), then bathe and lather up with hair conditioner. Next, apply liberal amounts of shaving gel, and use disposable razors to carefully shave off the hair. Use your hand to smooth down areas like the labia to get a good line. Women, ask your man for advice—they know more about this than you do. You could experiment with heart shapes or trimming initials if you don't want to go the whole way. Apply hypoallergenic lotion afterward to soothe it all down, which also helps when the hair's growing back.

Besides the risqué, using daily everyday objects to filthy effect is another good trick. For instance, use lipstick to draw around your penis, nipples, or labia. Have your partner lick and suck it off. That takes a lot of suction and you'll never hear the word "lipstick" together again without looking at each other knowingly.

You could also try wearing each other's underwear to work. For women, wearing a loose pair of boxers under a skirt let's the air circulate where it normally never gets to go and makes you feel more open in every sense of the word. For men, the feeling of constriction that comes from tight feminine panties under your business suit can be arousing—as well as all the other associations and images that will flash through your mind throughout the day.

Need help persuading your lover? Turn to IDEA 16, *Think kink.*

Try another idea...

Take this one step further and play around with cross-dressing. Wear each other's clothes in bed. You'll hate it or love it, but if you love it, you might be surprised at how much you love it. For men especially, breaking one of the last great heterosexual taboos (dressing as a woman) is a hugely liberating experience. Remember, no one knows but you two.

Need more inspiration? Go to a nude beach together, make a porn short, photograph each other nude, or have sex on the steps of your local library (make it a quickie!)—risky, but it will make you smile every time you drive to the supermarket.

And, of course, don't break the first rule of secrets. You don't tell. Ever.

"The real fountain of youth is to have a dirty mind."
JERRY HALL, actress and model

Defining idea...

How was
it for
you?

Q **Nothing you suggest appeals. Maybe we're not the secretive type. Anything else we can try?**

A *Of all the ideas in this book, this one has the most potential to be ridiculous. Sex makes us vulnerable, and that can make us feel foolish. If you're bereft of inspiration I suggest you think about someone you sit next to at work or an old friend. Then think of something sexual that if they knew about you'd die of mortification. You don't have to have done it—yet— you just have to be going red at the thought of them seeing you doing it. Got someone in mind? Well, there you go. That's the basis for a secret. Some things about our sex lives we wouldn't want anyone to know about, but we open ourselves up a lot by letting one other person share them. And that's sexy. A bit uncomfortable, but sexy, too.*

Q **I like having sexual secrets from my wife—it turns me on. I'm not really interested in sharing secrets with her though, it feels a little childish. Am I being selfish?**

A *It might be that you need to work on your sexual maturity a little. It seems like your wife is willing to share her secrets (which might be a big effort for her), so perhaps you need to try harder to do the same in return.*

43

Just say no

**There's saying no and there's saying no nicely. Two very
different things.**

Every relationship has its sexual deserts
when sex is off the table. Here's how to
negotiate your way through them so no one gets
too hurt.

Sometimes we simply want to say no. We might be tired. We might be feeling sad.
We might be preoccupied with something else. If your partner approaches you and
you feel ambivalent about having sex, my best advice is to go along with it for a
while and try to get yourself in the mood (with their help, of course). If, however,
you fail to rise onto that wave of lust, all you can do is gaze into their eyes tenderly
and say, "Sorry, it isn't working for me tonight, but I promise that tomorrow we'll
do the deed." Sex therapists pretty much agree that rejection is easier to take if
there's a definite date set for a retry. As a consolation prize and to give them the
human contact that we all crave (and which probably instigated their shuffle across
the bed in the first place), you could hold your partner while they masturbate to
orgasm. (And if you're not comfortable masturbating in front of each other, maybe
you ought to think about why not. It's a useful habit.)

Here's an idea for you... **If you and your partner haven't had sex for a month, sit down, look into his/her eyes, and ask why. The longer you go without sex, the easier it becomes to do without it. The more you do it, the more you'll want to.**

But what if you know that tomorrow you're not going to want to have sex either? What if this one's going to run and run? A genuine sexual desert, where it's been months and months and months, and you don't need so much to negotiate it as buy a map and a compass and start charting the unknown continent. First things first. Do you both want to emerge from your desert and find your oasis?

YES TO THE OASIS?

Is there a medical reason that one or both of you has lost interest in sex? Is it because one or both of you is having a midlife crisis? Deal with that and do the following.

NO TO THE OASIS

This one is tricky. You've lost interest in sex. You don't lust after your partner anymore. You can't be bothered to try. When they approach you, you simply don't want to do it.

Don't let sex be an ad hoc arrangement. Decide on a time when you're going to get physical and then do all you can to get yourself in the mood, such as a bath, delicious food, candles, or a chat. Enjoy each other. Don't expect mind-bending lust—mildly being up for it is good enough. If it's been a long time and you're a bit nervous about having sex, go back to basics. It doesn't matter what you do as long as you're physically close. Being physically close without having penetrative sex can eventually kick-start your libido. In fact, when you've been together for a while, you often need physical proximity to *start* feeling desire. In other words, you can't hang around waiting for an overwhelming wave of lust to wash over you or you'll wait a long time. Start having sex and let Mother Nature take her course.

If it's your partner who rejects your advances then read IDEA 12, *The love's there, but the lust's gone AWOL.*

Try another idea...

The bottom line is, if you can't be bothered to do all you can to get yourself and your partner in the mood for sex then you're a rotten lover. What's loving about a person who doesn't at

Can't be bothered with sex? Read IDEA 9, *Get over yourself.*

...and another

least try? This is brutal, but it's true. Perhaps you're right to take your lover's constancy for granted even when you're not putting out, trusting that they'll stick by you. But they're almost certain to get depressed and lose confidence—both traits are hell to live with and unlikely to endear them to you. Keeping your sex life going is as important for your mental health as theirs.

"Marriage, if it is to survive, must be treated as the beginning, not as the happy ending."
FEDERICO FELLINI

Defining idea...

How was it for you?

Q **I've been wandering the sexual desert following the birth of our children, but there's no oasis in sight. How much longer before the camel train arrives?**

A *There are usually two main problems here. The first is that either or both of you are simply not putting the relationship above other things, notably the kids. Time for some deep talking. Personally, I think that although parents would quite happily lay down their lives for their children, rarely are such sacrifices called for to keep them healthy and happy. If you're sacrificing your relationship for your kids, then that's your decision, but it's probably the wrong one.*

Q **I've told my partner a million times that to get in the mood I need time to chat, lots of foreplay, some buildup. So why does he persist in grabbing me when I'm unloading the dishwasher, muttering "want a quickie?" like a dirty old man and then getting huffy when I tell him to kiss off?**

A *He probably hates having to go through your proscribed dance of seduction. This isn't all about sex. He's resentful that you get to decide when and how you'll have sex. There's a power struggle between you two that's being enacted over the battleground that is your dishwasher. Your partner may just yearn for a quickie and not know how to ask you for one. Would it be the end of the world if you succumbed? Of course, if sometimes you do succumb, then there's nothing complicated or psychological going on at all. He's just taking a chance on the principle that if one time out of fifty you say yes, he might get lucky again.*

44

It's not all in your mind

If you've lost interest in sex, it may be time to see your doctor.

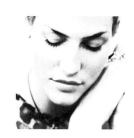

Our bodies affect our libido much more than we'd care to admit.

It's an odd person that goes through life with the same level of sexual vigor. Our income, lifestyle, confidence levels, and any medication we've been prescribed by our doctors all affect how much desire we feel. But the big daddy that affects our libido is a hormonal change. Hormones determine so much about our lives, from how attractive we look (ovulating women get better looking) to the sorts of films we want to watch (new parents of both sexes have trouble with war movies).

This is why it's so odd that when we lose interest in sex we don't head straight to the doctor for a checkup. What's even odder is how little use most of our doctors are if we actually do get there. I'm not knocking doctors, but they have limited resources and these tend to be focused on patients with cancer rather than those who only feel like sex once a month. So you'll have to do a lot of medical research yourself if you feel that your health is standing in the way of your love life. The Internet is a wonderful thing; just don't start sending away for things that promise to make your penis bigger.

Here's an
idea for
you... **A lack of desire is one of the major symptoms of depression. It's also a side effect of some antidepressant drugs. What we call a catch-22. In cases of mild to moderate depression, exercise has been shown to be as effective as medication and might be well worth trying seriously.**

We have very limited space, but this chapter is going to give you a few ideas to start you off on your own road to discovery vis-à-vis your body and provide you with some key words to type into the search engine. "I want to have sex more" isn't a great thing to let Google know about.

ARE YOU TAKING ANY MEDICATION?

If you are, you really do need to speak to your doctor. Many different kinds of medication, including those for heart conditions and depression, can lower your libido. Some forms of the contraceptive pill also make you less interested in sex. Your doctor may be able to change your prescription, but she won't be able to do that if you don't tell her there's a problem in the first place.

YOU'VE HAD A KID

The theory is that women lose interest in sex so that they can concentrate on one baby's survival before conceiving another. My theory is that it's their own survival they're concerned about. Don't believe the books that tell you recovery only takes six weeks; but it doesn't take two years either. Having said that, many women aren't interested in sex for literally years after giving birth—a weird physical and psychological inertia takes over. Eventually, you've just got to get back in the saddle and use every trick to rebuild your libido from the ground up.

If you're a man who's lost interest big-time since your child's been born, two things: You could be a terrific bonder producing tons of a hormone that actually suppresses testosterone in new fathers, making you happy to hang around the metaphorical campfire with your missus and the little one rather than, say, popping into the cave next door for some variety. In which case, your libido will come back. Alternatively, you could have deep-rooted psychological hang-ups along the Madonna/whore axis. In which case, you need therapy.

Read IDEA 49, *Dealing with burnout*. The mind can have a profound effect on the body. Maybe your state of mind is affecting yours.

Try another idea...

YOU'RE OF A CERTAIN AGE

By this, I mean anything from about thirty-five on. For women, that's when the perimenopause kicks in—the period (no pun intended) leading up to menopause proper. Your hormonal balance alters and although some women experience nothing at all, others are forgetful, moody, irritable, and, of course, less interested in sex. Your doctor may be able to prescribe HRT depending on your hormonal levels, but you may not be happy with this. There are a host of herbal remedies that can help maintain libido in the years up to and following menopause. Try black cohosh and red clover.

"I once made love for an hour and fifteen minutes. But it was the night the clocks were set ahead."
GARY SHANDLING, comedian

Defining idea...

How was it for you?

Q   Do men have a male menopause?

A   *It seems that some do—the so-called andropause. So far, it's not been proven, but what has been found is that some men do respond to testosterone medication and regain their lust along with their love for life.*

Q   Would Viagra help me get my libido back?

A   *It might, but Viagra isn't completely without problems. One of the most obvious problems is that in a relationship where a man has had problems with arousal, his sudden priapic and demanding new persona can cause havoc. Read up on all the pros and cons and discuss it with your partner and doctor beforehand.*

Q   I've put on a lot of weight and thought that was the reason I wasn't interested in sex.

A   *It could be, but the weight gain might be a symptom of a condition that is robbing you of sexual desire. Low thyroid hormones is one possibility. So is diabetes or menopause. Go to your doctor for a checkup and make sure you discuss your low libido as well as your weight gain.*

Pressure—it's not a dirty word

Or rather, if you're doing it right, it can be.

For most, sex is the main course of lovemaking. Oh, OK, for most, sex is more of a quick snack. But for times when (to push the meal metaphor to the limit) you want to feast on a banquet of love, there is massage.

You don't need to be self-conscious about massaging each other. It doesn't have to be of a professional standard because what you lack in technique you can more than make up for by what is called "loving intention"; your total focus on your partner's relaxation and pleasure will do lots of good.

First, select your oil. You can buy massage oils premixed or create your own blend by adding eight to ten drops of oil (or a mixture of oils) to three dessertspoons of a base oil such as almond. Good oils for sensual massage are geranium, which is uplifting and grounding; lavender, which is relaxing and soothing; sandalwood, which is warming and encouraging; and ylang ylang, which is sensual and erotic. Burning the same combination of oils as you massage will heighten the experience for your lover.

Here's an idea for you...

Maintain skin-to-skin contact throughout the massage. Cup one hand on your lover's back while you pour more oil so that the back of your hand maintains this contact.

Choose a warm, comfortable place in your home. Put on some gentle music and lower the lights. Take a bath or shower together. The masseur (or masseuse) should dress in light comfortable clothes and make their lover comfortable lying on their front.

Take some oil—and you should have liberal amounts on hand—and warm it between your palms. Then start working the oil into your partner's back. Use firm gliding strokes over the large muscles of the shoulder blades, then work down the sides to the base of the spine and then work upward using the balls of your thumbs to apply pressure on either side of the spine. The secret of applying pressure is to channel the strength of your body through the balls of your thumbs. Lean into your lover's body but apply pressure only to the meaty parts of the body (but not the belly). Don't apply pressure on hard bony areas.

Continue with sweeping movements alternated by gentle pressure across the back, buttocks, and the back of legs. Use long strokes along the arms and gently pull at each finger in turn. Try different pressures. Use fists to apply heavier kneading movements to the buttocks. Apply very light blows across the back. Then alternate with gentle fingertip stroking.

Don't worry about your technique, just concentrate on your lover's body and giving it pleasure. Ask for a little feedback. For example, does your partner want a gentler or firmer stroke? But don't talk too much. Allow your partner to relax into the massage.

Ask your partner to turn over. Holding their head steady with your knees and massaging their face is particularly relaxing. Don't apply heavy pressure to the stomach. Brush but don't directly touch their genitals—the oils may irritate sensitive areas. Anyway, the point is to build sensual pleasure for you both, not necessarily to move onto sex. Judge how your partner feels. Are they giving the impression that this is turning them on? Or is it so relaxing that they want to curl up in your arms and sleep? If you're not sure, ask them, and don't let your wishes come through either way. Making it clear you expect sex in return for giving a massage isn't considered good taste.

Explore your potential for touch in IDEA 13, *Touchy-feely*.

Try another idea...

SHORTCUT TO BLISS

If you don't have the time to indulge in a full body treat, give a foot massage instead.

Bathe your lover's feet. A few drops of peppermint oil in a basin refresh instantly and keeps things fresh for you. Then ask them to sit while you kneel at their feet, with a towel over your knees to cradle each foot in turn. Massage oil over one foot. Apply pressure through your thumbs systematically all over the soles of the feet. Concentrate particularly on the fleshy parts of each toe in turn and gently pull and rotate each one. If you're feeling particularly loving, wipe the oil from your lover's nails and give them a pedicure (men, too). Men, painting your lover's toenails means she remembers your heavenly foot massage every time she catches sight of her tootsies—an easy way of garnering Brownie points.

"To lovers, touch is metamorphosis. All the parts of their bodies seem to change, and seem to become something different and better."
JOHN CHEEVER, writer

Defining idea...

How was it for you?

Q We don't often have time for the whole nine yards. Any shortcuts?

A *You can use acupressure in seconds during sex to heighten your lover's sexual pleasure. The ancient Chinese teach that pressing acupressure points is like a concentrated massage, releasing tension and building pleasure. One spot directly above the penis or clitoris and one on each side activates points that are linked to increasing sexual energy and by pressing these you arouse your lover faster. There's another series of three points in the front of the thighs in the crease where the pubis meets the thigh. Pressing there heightens sensitivity, especially when you're giving oral sex. Finally, imagine a line drawn between the pubic area and the hip bone on each side. Pressing along "the crease" there increases pleasurable feelings in the genitals. Press firmly and relax—don't press any of these points for much more than a couple of minutes at a time.*

Q I find that receiving a massage tickles and it's distracting. Any advice?

A *Your lover needs to exert more pressure. Ask them to lean in harder. Give them feedback until you receive the level of pressure you want.*

Q Why don't I like giving massages? I don't like receiving it much, either...

A *There could be all sorts of reasons for this, but let's cut to the chase—a possible solution. Perhaps you feel embarrassed. Try using the god/goddess or priest/priestess fantasy. If you're receiving a massage, you're the god/goddess and it's the greatest pleasure and honor for your priest/priestess to be serving you. Reverse this if you're the priest or priestess serving the deity. Get out of your head and concentrate on the physical.*

Wait. We said wait!

Delay orgasm—aka "peaking"—and you'll know the true meaning of "climb every mountain."

Is there a woman alive who, on approaching the big "O," hasn't muttered, "Don't stop, for God's sake, don't stop"? A woman's biggest fear is that with the finish line in sight, he changes his stroke, everything goes wrong, and she doesn't make it.

So, when a woman feels herself on the edge of an orgasm she'll rush her way there. It's hard-earned and she wants it now. But here's another way for her to do it. On the point of orgasm, she could slow down, relax, breathe deeply, wait a moment or so, and then let the tension build again. Experiment with this (either with your partner or while masturbating) to discover how long you have to stop–start, stop–start to get the most explosive orgasms. When you do allow yourself to come, clenching buttocks and inner thighs, deep breathing, and pressing down just above your pubic bone all increase blood flow, which keeps the sensation going.

Here's an idea for you... **Play a game where you oil each other and try to give your mate an orgasm with a different part of your body from usual. (Boob job, anyone?)**

NOT JUST FOR THE GIRLS

Advocates of all ways Eastern recommend "injaculation," a way that men can experience multiple orgasms by "coming" without ejaculation. This means he can go again right away, experience multiple bliss, and, of course, keep going longer.

Try another idea... **Combine this with what you read in IDEA 45, *Pressure—it's not a dirty word.***

How to do it? Business as usual until just before the point of "no return." Then swiftly, either you or your partner applies circular (quite heavy) pressure to your perineum, the space midway between your anus and the root of your penis. This causes pressure on the urethra and will stop you ejaculating, although you should still experience a deeply pleasurable, not to say mind-boggling, sensation. And you should still be hard—ready to play again should the mood take you. And it will, of course.

Some men love this. Some don't. One who doesn't is Grant Stoddard, who is quoted in *The Big Bang* by Em & Lo: "The buildup to the orgasm was momentarily more intense than usual. I realized I could go right away again and did until I got bored and a bit depressed. The real shocker came when I went to the bathroom to find that my pee had more head on it than a pint of Guinness. In other words, I'd just come in my bladder. And that's f**ked up."

Defining idea... **"Made a hell of a discovery the other night. Eyelashes on the clit...can blink her off in no time."**
DAN JENKINS, writer

But worth a try.

Q What about women's multiple orgasms?

A   *Theoretically, if a woman can come once, she can come multiple times. It's commonly believed that straight after a woman has come, she can't bear to have her clitoris touched. Sometimes true, but not always. Experiment with different techniques during masturbation. Swap to a different hand motion after you've come, or if you're using a vibrator try a different hot spot. Keep stimulation constant, but varied. Once you have the hang of that, masturbate to orgasm and stop masturbating completely after the first orgasm. Wait thirty seconds and then apply the same stimulation to the clitoris again. Shorten the waiting period until you can keep the stimulation at constant without it being uncomfortable, and experience orgasm after orgasm rolling over you.*

Q Is there any way we can practice peaking together?

A   *You can go for the blended orgasm. This means applying stimulation at different pleasure points so excitement mounts. He can stimulate her G-spot, her clitoris, and her perineum one after another in rotation. She can stimulate the head of his penis, the shaft, and the prostate in rotation. This takes time, but should result in a long, delayed, and sweeter blend of intense pleasure and melting ecstasy when you come.*

How was it for you?

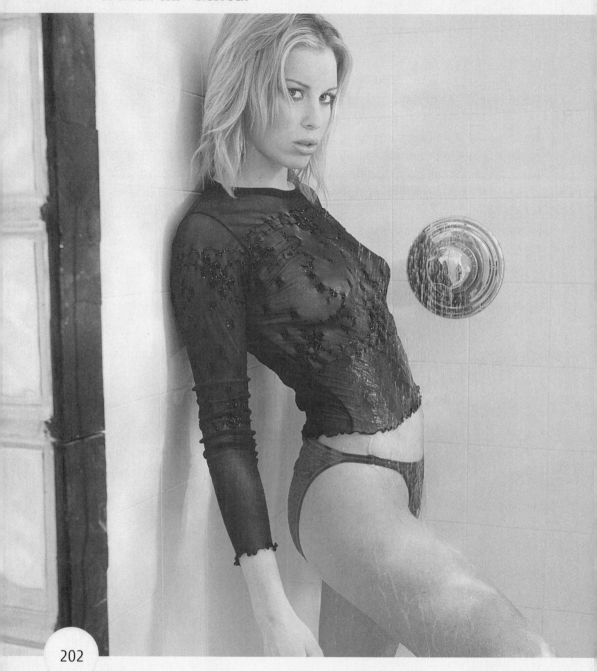

Developing sexual mystique

Yes, it's possible. Even if you've shared a bathroom for years.

Last night I had a moment of despair. I walked by a bar where I overheard a man saying to his (male) companion, "So guess. How many shots did the Heat take during the game last night?"

Admittedly, even his friend looked bored, but I thought, "Here I am, working at building more understanding between the sexes in my own small way. And it's a total waste of time. Men and women? Different species. What's the point?"

Then my natural Pollyanna spirit kicked in, "Differences—you know what? They're a Good Thing. In fact, if you want to keep your love life hot, they're an Essential Thing. To continue desiring your partner and to have them continue desiring you, you need a little distance between you, a little mystery, a little wildness in your soul."

And if that doesn't come naturally, you need to work at it.

Here's an idea for you... **In a nutshell, make it a habit that one night a week you do your own thing, no matter how busy you are. Remember, spending too much time inside together is terrible for your love life.**

"Males and females are different," says relationship counselor Paula Hall. "And we've known since the '60s that if a couple wants a stable relationship, it's worth working at maintaining that difference. It's what keeps the electric buzz between them." She points out that studies by psychologists have already picked up on the dangers of becoming too alike. "We call it 'enmeshment,' when couples become too similar," says Hall. "It's been known for a long time that it can have a detrimental impact on sexual desire."

You probably think it's cozy that you share the same interests, friends, hopes, dreams, taste in soft furnishings. So it is. Congratulations. You're terrific mates. And carry on regardless if you want a great relationship without particularly exciting, or indeed plentiful, sex. However, if you want sex that makes your toes curl, you need a little separateness to keep desire alive.

You can be all things to a partner, but not to a lover. They cannot be all things to you.

There's an art to this. One woman I interviewed made a point of always being just a little bit cool with her husband every three or four months or so. "Nothing serious," she said, "I'd just switch off from him for a while. Seem a little bit less easily pleased. A bit more interested in talking to my friends on the phone. Lock myself in the bathroom. Submerge myself in a book. Really trivial stuff. Worked like a charm. Within a week, he'd be suggesting weekends away in Paris and voluntarily arranging babysitting so we could go out to dinner." (I can't resist the opportunity here to remind men of the huge aphrodisiac potential in occasionally arranging for a babysitter. In most relationships, whether or not the woman works from home or not, she does the babysitting stuff—it's so damn nice when your partner works it out for once, as it's such a clear signal that you want to spend some time with her. Try it.)

All this withdrawing interest sounds suspiciously like game-playing—and you know what, it is! You can fake it a little bit like my interviewee, but it doesn't always work. What does always work is if both partners do it for real—keep interested in life, stay full of vim and vigor for other projects, remain engaged with people outside of their relationship, and be passionate about the world. Then, and here is the important part, they bring that energy home and translate it into passion for each other. They do that by talking about their lives with such enthusiasm that their partners can't help getting a kick out of their enthusiasm, charm, intelligence, and all-around top-quality personality.

Read IDEA 22, *Sexual confidence*, for ideas on building self-esteem and individuality.

Try another idea...

"*An absence, the declining of an invitation to dinner, an unintentional, unconscious harshness are of more service than all the cosmetics and fine clothes in the world.*"
MARCEL PROUST

Defining idea...

THE LEAST YOU NEED TO DO...

Relationship psychologist Susan Quilliam points out that there are straightforward ways of making sure your relationship doesn't sink into the mire of "enmeshment."

Rule 1. All couples fall into a pattern of doing the same thing and being scared to suggest anything new because "we don't do that." But if you want to do something different, suggest it anyway. Don't argue if they say no. The point has been made. You've reinforced in both your minds that you're different individuals.

Rule 2. Support your partner as much as possible when they're trying to be an individual. Don't dismiss new ideas and interests without thinking them through carefully.

Rule 3. Be yourself. Don't take on his or her interests and hobbies unless they genuinely interest you, too. We're equal but we're not the same.

Q   My partner's interest is hours spent in Internet chat rooms. What's gone wrong?

How was it for you?

A   *You're insecure in your relationship for some reason and probably for a very good reason. Whatever your partner chooses to do on their own that you view as a threat—chat rooms, lap dancing, drinking, Smurf collecting—isn't a problem in itself. It's the fact that you perceive it as a threat that's the problem. Yours is not a happy ship or your partner would stop or significantly cut down on the chat rooms when you expressed discomfort. A little bit of mystery only works to spice up healthy, functional relationships, and yours isn't. Time to start talking.*

Q   I tried being a bit withdrawn, but he didn't notice. Any ideas what I should try next?

A   *I'd guess that he's the one who proffers the cheek to be kissed and you're the one always doing the kissing. It's tough for kissers because they're genuinely focused on their mates pretty much to the detriment of everything else and it's hard to fake indifference. He knows what you're trying to do and kind of likes it. He'll ignore you even more—sorry, but that's the nature of the push-pull, passive-aggressive relationship you've formed. Until now it's worked for you, but maybe you now want something different. The solution for you is the solution for all of us when we want to change our relationships. Stop thinking about his reactions, expect nothing different from him, and concentrate on you. Reintroduce passion into your own life. You've gone beyond the stage of playing games. It's time to get real about your life. If he's the only thing that really gets your juices going, change that fast.*

207

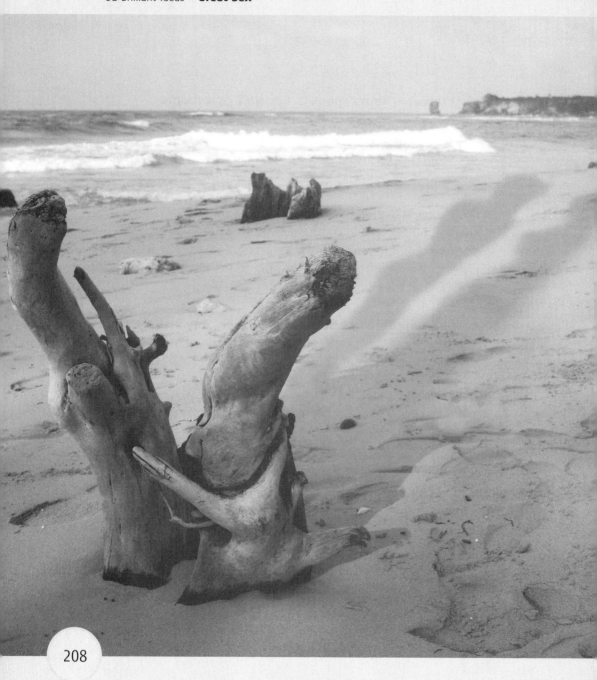

See things differently

Give yourself a real eye-opener.

Explore voyeurism and exhibitionism and bring a completely new forbidden edge to your love life.

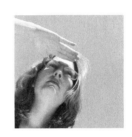

The following fantasy role-plays depend on our love of looking and our love of being watched. Use these as a starting point to begin exploring your own voyeuristic or exhibitionistic fantasies—nearly all of us are turned on by one, and usually both. If you'd like to strip, but are too shy, then the second "Peeping Tom" fantasy is a good place to start. You can start dropping clothes without feeling self-conscious, as you're not doing it (ostensibly) for an audience.

IMAGINE...

Your partner comes home to find the house lit by candles. You lead them to the bathroom where there is a scented bath waiting. You undress, blindfold, and wash them. You don't let them do anything for themselves. Then you lead them to the bedroom, also lit only by candles, where there's a huge mirror propped to give a

It can be very erotic to take turns ordering each other to perform. Some people love being ordered to strip or perform from the outset. Others hate it and bristle when their partner tells them what to do, even if it's done in an encouraging way. So be sensitive, as for one or both of you it may have to be a natural development.

great reflection of the bed or, if that's not possible, the floor covered in cushions and quilts. Remove the blindfold and then make love, staring at yourself in the mirror, holding your lover's gaze. Try half closing your eyes so that you can fantasize that it isn't you, but another couple writhing inches away from you—accomplices at an orgy. Go one step further and imagine that the couple in the mirror are another couple that you're observing—to help the illusion, wear corsets, wigs, a new pair of heels, etc.

IMAGINE...

In the morning, you give your partner explicit written instructions of what you want them to do and at what hour you want them to start. At ten minutes before the appointed hour, you go to your bedroom, move clothes out of your closet into the spare room, place a chair in the closet, and sit inside it with the door open a crack so you can see the bed. Your partner arrives in the bedroom. He or she follows the instructions you gave them earlier. They slowly begin to get ready for bed. If they get into it, this can be a long tease. They pass in and out of your field of vision, shedding clothes; trying on different clothes, lingerie, or nightwear, examining their reflection; massaging in oils and creams before bed; phoning a friend and idly touching themselves as they talk; wandering out of the room to get themselves a drink. They are seemingly oblivious to your presence. Eventually, they take up the position that you've stipulated and, still "unaware" that you're there, they give serious attention to bringing themselves off in front of your eager gaze.

IMAGINE...

You are the stars of a live porn show. You have a clearly defined stage area (either your bed or a rug on your living room floor, brightly lit with spotlights). You both dress and prepare yourselves in your "dressing room." You can hear the pounding music in the background that you'll perform to and (imagine) the applause and excitement emanating from the audience. You take up position on your stage and begin to strip each other. Remember, everyone in the club has to see every detail and every act is exaggerated to give a maximum eyeful to the people standing, craning at the back. Massage oil into each other's bodies. When you start to have sex, remember this— it's a show. Everything has to be seen. Your audience loves it, and you can feel the tense silence as they watch you strip and the growing excitement as the sex becomes more explicit, more frenzied. You two get more excited, louder, more vocal, urging each other on verbally. When he comes, it should be over her body— the so-called "money shot" beloved of porn films.

Turn to IDEA 23, *What you see...*, for more on visual arousal.

Try another idea...

"There are only two guidelines for good sex: 'Don't do anything you don't really enjoy' and 'find out your partner's needs and don't balk at them if you can help it.' "
DR. ALEX COMFORT, author of *The Joy of Sex*

Defining idea...

How was
it for
you?

Q   Does this have to be so complicated?

A   *It doesn't have to be. Park your car in a remote spot and play at being teenagers again. Taking risks in public is something that tends to diminish when we've been together for a while, which is a shame because although these risks may be uncomfortable, they'll make you feel far more daring than when you genuinely were a teenager. OK, you're respectable pillars of the community now, but you can still do it somewhere where you could be overlooked without taking much of a risk of it actually happening. Just thinking that you're being watched is a great turn-on.*

Q   We want to film ourselves having sex. Where do we begin?

A   *If one of you is shy, play around with the last fantasy role-play in this idea. It's only one step away from setting up your camcorder while pretending to be porn stars. You'll want the lights on—fumbling in the dark feels good, but looks lousy (which is why the above fantasy is a good starter because the spotlit "stage" gets you used to performing in bright lights). You want the tripod fixed.*

49

Dealing with burnout

That's what we call it when you don't want sex and you just don't care. In fact, you don't seem to care about much of anything at all.

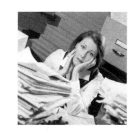

How do you know when you're dealing with burnout?

PROBLEM: TOO MANY PEOPLE WANT A PIECE OF YOU

Solution: Set boundaries and cut down on commitments

People who don't set boundaries often end up playing out their frustrations in the bedroom: "You don't give me what I need, so you won't get what you need." This is equally true for the woman who withdraws sex as the man who, although he wants sex, isn't affectionate because he feels overburdened with responsibility. When you're too tired for sex or to give your partner what they need to feel good, the answer is to spend time cutting loose from all commitment. Time alone gives you a sense of balance and renewal, which can give you more energy.

How do you find that time? By setting boundaries. Here's what Dr. Alan Altman says in his book *Making Love the Way We Used To, or Better*: "You need to genuinely believe the following: You have needs. Those needs are as important as other people's needs. You can help others, but you do not have to be everyone's answer to everything. Sometimes saying no is a gift to the other person, who grows and becomes stronger by learning more self-reliance."

Here's an idea for you...

Read books that thrilled you in your teens. Read books that make you horny. Listen to music that makes you feel sexual (or free, romantic, wild, independent). It could be Bruce Springsteen, Van Morrison, or Morrissey. Whatever, if it rocks your boat then play it loud and play it often. Dance around your bedroom.

PROBLEM: YOU'RE BORED WITH LIFE

Solution: Rediscover your passion and revel in pleasure

My definition of a midlife crisis is pretty loose. It goes like this. You're aged anything from thirty-two upward and you suddenly start feeling terribly, terribly scared. You're scared you've made mistakes. You're scared you haven't made enough mistakes. You're scared you'll be driving a beater car for the rest of your life. You're scared of your belly, more specifically the rate at which it's growing. These all amount to the same thing. You're scared of death.

Understandably, fear of death translates into a dissatisfaction with your version of the most life-affirming activity we've got—sex. And, more specifically, the partner you've chosen to have sex with. I'm not just talking about men here. What's fueling the Viagra explosion is a whole raft of fifty-something women who are waking up and going, "You know what, I'm bored of faking orgasms. Call this a sex life? I don't." This is frightening the bejesus out of fifty-something men and they're hoping Viagra is the answer.

Anyway, I digress. The point is, if you're bored with having sex with your partner but you still love them, you have to talk instead of repeatedly saying no. Tell your partner honestly, "I'm worried. I'm fed up with

IDEA 44, *It's not all in your mind*, has more on the physical and mental obstacles to a great sex life.

Try another idea...

everything. I don't have juice for anything much, and with your help I want to get back my va-va-voom." Then you can negotiate more time for yourself, more vacations together, the purchase of a nice big vibrator, dressing up as Santa Claus. Whatever it takes to get more pleasure into your life, because pleasure is the only cure for a midlife crisis and all other forms of burnout. Your partner might not like some of your ideas—they're never going to think that a Harley Davidson is a great idea and they're certainly not going to warm to the leather chaps. But if yours is a good healthy relationship then they'll live with whatever it takes to return you to the happy love bunny you were of yore. Unless, of course, it threatens them or the relationship, in which case you don't have a healthy relationship and you need the sort of help that's outside the scope of this idea. Good luck with the therapy.

"Sex without love is an empty experience, but, as empty experiences go, it's one of the best."
WOODY ALLEN

Defining idea...

How was
it for
you?

**Q   I hate my job. I'm exhausted, but there's no way I can cut down on
my workload. What can I do?**

A   *It's impossible to get in touch with your inner sex god or goddess if you're
totally stressed out and exhausted. David Deida says that working too hard
can be detrimental to some relationships, especially for women, and that
"common financial needs have replaced commitment and desire as the
motivating forces in many relationships." I want to disagree with him,
especially about the emphasis on women. But I can't. Everywhere I see
many women and some men who are tired and confused. Who can argue
with the fact that "common financial needs" have hijacked many couples'
lives, including yours? Lack of interest in sex is only one of your problems.
Anger, resentment, and disappointment are all probably waving their hands
to be noticed, too. But unless you're on absolute subsistence, then you
have choices. You're going to have to have constructive, creative discussions
with your partner about exactly what you need to get happy and stay that
way.*

**Q   Exactly what do you mean by getting more pleasure into my life?
If I knew how, I would.**

A   *The surest route to pleasure and passion is to get creative. Make a habit of
expressing what you really think and feel. There are a million ways to do
this—organizing a pub quiz can be creative if you want it to be. I can't tell
you what makes you passionate or gives you pleasure. Some spiritual types
would say that's what we're on the planet to discover. You either pursue
your potential for creativity, passion, and pleasure or you don't. It's your call.*

50

Dream time

Sexual fantasy—a shortcut to great sex.

Read on if your response was,
"Who's got the time?"

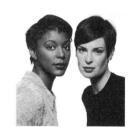

Somebody once said that sexual fantasy was the "thinking man's television," and they weren't kidding. Hours of entertainment and you don't even have to leave your sofa to enjoy it. If you get up off your butt and take your fantasies into the bedroom, they'll give you explosive orgasms, too. What goes on in your mind is as important as what's going on around your genitals. However, just like talking dirty, it has to be your own "script." Many people read the lists of top male fantasies or top female fantasies (usually both headed by lesbian sex) and think "bull." I'm not being judgmental. If you're a woman who thinks about two women getting it on and this drives you over the edge, terrific. But if it doesn't, you shouldn't give up finding out what does. Men tend to have more access to porn, and that hot-wires their fantasies and preferences pretty early on. Women don't usually have this advantage and by the time they get to adulthood are often too busy unloading the dishwasher to care. But bear with me. Even if sexual fantasy isn't a big part of your life right now, it's a habit well worth getting into.

WHY?

Sexual fantasy increases your libido. The more you think about sex, the more you want it. Plus, just a glimmer of the thought of your fantasy during sex will increase your pleasure a hundredfold and if you're a woman it'll make orgasm faster (if

Here's an idea for you...

Once you've discovered fantasyland, up the dirtiness quotient. The true power of fantasy lies in forbidden thoughts, so try thinking of some real extremes. Remember, this has nothing to do with who you are in real life.

Defining idea...

"I caused my husband's heart attack. In the middle of lovemaking, I took the paper bag off my head. He dropped the Polaroid and keeled over and so did the hooker. It would have taken me half an hour to untie myself and call the paramedics, but fortunately the Great Dane could dial."
JOAN RIVERS

you're a guy, more enjoyable). Also, a strong fantasy life is invaluable for those times when your partner reaches for you and you're not sure if you can be bothered. Letting your favorite fantasy tickle your imagination for a second or two can be the deciding factor as to whether you respond with alacrity or shrug them off. My view is that happier relationships result when the response is the former.

WHAT?

A friend once recounted some of her dreams to me, "I fantasize about having two men at one time or having sex with someone else while my boyfriend watches. I fantasize about getting oral sex from under the table at a restaurant or about being screwed during a gynecological exam. Usually I don't have time to make an elaborate fantasy during sex, but conjuring up any one of these quick images will do."

Your fantasy might be something that you won't find on a list of "top fantasies." For instance, there's some evidence that in the post-feminist age, many women love the idea of homosexual sex—but with men, not women. A gay man means a good body and a challenge—just the sort of thing a feisty woman would enjoy fantasizing about. (Hmm . . . perhaps that's Madonna's thing.) But women willing to admit to it are rare. Hell, women even realizing that thinking about gay men could do it for them are rare. As with most things to do with sex, gender politics probably come into it. Women aren't sexually liberated enough to talk about a fantasy that doesn't turn straight men on. In

For inspiration look to IDEA 51, *Fantasy destinations.*

Try another idea…

fact, since erect dicks are in the equation, it'll probably threaten them. This could be one reason why women don't fantasize as much—their fantasies don't appear on any of those lists so they think they're weird and give up on them. If none of the traditional female fantasies ring your bell, then read *My Secret Garden*, *Women on Top*, or *Men in Love* by Nancy Friday—an absolute eye-opener (and a turn-on) for both sexes.

HOW?

You can either be in the fantasy, or observe your fantasy as you would a film. Start telling yourself a story. A story where you're the hero/heroine—as gorgeous as you like. An American comic had a great gag, "When I fantasize, *I'm* someone else." And although it's meant to be funny, he's got it nailed: You can be the person you'd like to be.

Your fantasy can be filled with people you know really well or people you glimpsed on a bus twenty years ago, and again they can be idealized versions—more exciting, demanding, inventive. Think in detail. Tell yourself these stories while masturbating. Imagine hands grasping, tongues licking, words being whispered. (You don't need the whole story when you're making love, just a flash of a detailed scene.) It takes practice.

"I say to men, 'OK, pretend you're a burglar and you break in and throw me down on the bed and make me suck your cock.' And they're horrified. 'No, no, it would degrade you.' Exactly. Degrade me when I ask you to."
LISA PALAC, writer

Defining idea…

219

How was
it for
you?

Q My fantasies are no problem, but they're very raunchy. Should I share them?

A Couples are always being exhorted to share fantasies, and this can be a big mistake. Men know this. I always remember the shock of asking the most conventional boyfriend I ever had to tell me what he fantasized about and he blithely and immediately answered "golden showers." I was stunned into silence. Later, intrigued, I asked him more. Either my boyfriend was teasing me on or didn't want to ever go there in reality (me too, if I'm being honest), as he clammed up. Some sharing will definitely enhance your lovemaking, but maybe it would be better to keep the one about defecating nuns to yourself.

Q Can you give me some inspiration?

A Both sexes fantasize about sex with a stranger. Women get off on the element of being forced—to strip, to have sex with one or multiple men. Often these fantasies get exotic—the sultan and the harem, the plundering pirate. Another version is the casting couch or the job interview where you have to give sex to get ahead in your career. Showing off is big for women—stripping or lap dancing—and the "seducing a virgin" works for both sexes. Women often imagine having to teach one or many young men how to pleasure a woman. And, of course, there's lesbian sex and being watched secretly. Another big favorite is sex with someone forbidden—your partner's best friend rather than your mother-in-law, obviously. Or maybe not... There I go, being judgmental.

dream

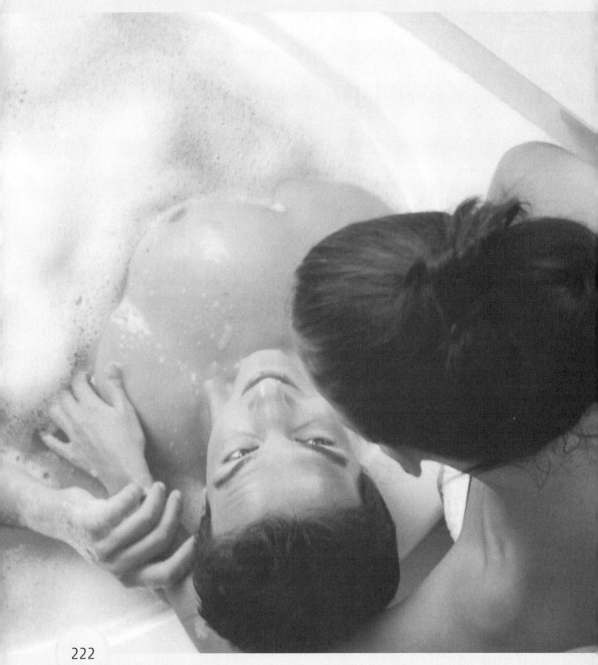

51

Fantasy destinations

Great places to have sex—and you don't have to get a babysitter.

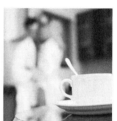

Doing it differently is part of the foundation for constantly exciting sex. Every so often, make one of your dates an at-home soiree. Decide on your fantasy destination—use your imagination and introduce as much role-play as you feel comfortable with.

A fantasy destination is a good laugh. It's a cheap game and it gets your creative juices flowing. How many classic/cliched love scenes can you reenact without leaving your house? Here are some to get you going:

TOP FIVE FANTASY DESTINATIONS

The alpine lodge in a blizzard (your living room)
It's winter. Deep winter. You are two climbers who've had to take shelter in a remote log cabin, cut off from the rest of the human race and locked in by a

Here's an idea for you...

Plan your fantasy trip carefully. Take time to run through the scenario in your mind and write your own script (mentally). Unless you're both great at improvization and have a bit of a competitive streak, then it will typically take two or three fantasy destinations for you to get a grip on it.

blizzard. You have no electricity, little food, but luckily lots of brandy. You spread a blanket in front of the log fire, light a couple of candles, and sip at your brandy. Outside the wind is howling. Your fellow climber is looking more attractive by the minute. Soon it seems a very good idea to get under the blanket (or better still, into a very cozy sleeping bag) and huddle together for warmth...

Working late at the office (your kitchen)

One of you is the boss. The boss has very high standards and expects a great deal from their assistant. The assistant is working late one night (at your kitchen table posing as a desk), bent over their work with only a desk lamp for illumination. Suddenly, the boss strides in and throws a sheaf of papers at the hapless assistant's head and lets loose with a stream of invective along the lines of, "This is garbage. If you want to keep your job, you're going to have to be punished until you do it better." The hapless assistant is tied up to a chair while the boss begins to undress the assistant and himself and hisses, "You'd like to touch me, but you're so incompetent you wouldn't know what to do with it." The boss then proceeds to show the assistant how it should be done, ordering the assistant to help make amends for past mistakes.

The sauna (your bathroom)

It's very hot and steamy (thanks to your shower being on full). So steamy that at first you don't see that someone else is sharing the sauna with you. Then you notice a figure sitting close by wrapped in a white towel. You smile uncertainly then shut your eyes and relax, letting the steam overwhelm you. You open your eyes. Your companion is staring at you. Their towel falls open. Everyone is supposed to wear swimsuits but you never do, and they obviously don't either. You're embarrassed. Should you point out that their towel has slipped or let your own slip a little, too...?

Still not convinced? For some inspiration read IDEA 14, Surprise!

Try another idea...

Camping out (your yard, in summer)

You and a friend have gone on a vacation walking in the hills. After a long day, you set up camp (or settle under the stars in your sleeping bags) in the middle of nowhere. You switch on a flashlight, have some dinner, share some jokes, drink some wine, play a game of cards. Before you know it, the game of cards has turned into a strip version of the game and things get very friendly in your tent (or, if you're unperturbed by the neighbors, under the stars)...

Murder in the dark (your house, with the lights off)

You're both guests at a country house party. A fellow guest has suggested a game of murder in the dark. One of you goes off to hide somewhere in the dark silent house. One of you is the murderer who stealthily hunts them down, getting closer and closer. But when the murderer finds the victim, there's another surprise for both of them...

"The most romantic thing a woman ever said to me in bed was, 'Are you sure you're not a cop?'"
LARRY BROWN, comedian

Defining idea...

How was
it for
you?

Q **I'm game, but my partner thinks the whole thing is ridiculous. Any more tips?**

A *Pick one of the scenarios that involves minimal role-playing. Out of the above, that's the camping one. If they absolutely refuse to have sex in a tent in your backyard under cover of darkness, you may have to give up on this one. However, you can try talking about fantasy situations in the privacy of your own bed, as just talking fantasy can be a terrific boost to your love life.*

Q **We tried the tent in the yard, but by the time we'd put it up it was hard to get in character. How do we stop the organizing from getting in the way?**

A *Admittedly, figuring it out together can be a little off-putting. It's more fun if you take turns being the "party coordinator" responsible for gathering the props, decorating the room if necessary, organizing outfits if appropriate, and making sure any food or alcohol that's required are on tap. Leave a note explaining the scenario, with any clothes you want your lover to wear, laid out on the bed.*

52

Are you sexually mature?

It is big and it is clever.

I've got a theory about what happens when couples are no longer connecting sexually. That theory goes something like this...

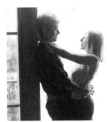

Men and women may enjoy casual sex in much the same way, but when it comes to the long haul—the big relationship where the expectations and desire of each partner is that it lasts for the foreseeable future—different attitudes toward what constitutes closeness can develop over the years. I'm going to generalize like crazy, so you two might not conform to this pattern, but on the whole women seem to show their love through emotional closeness and need their partner to show them that he loves them through emotional closeness—talking, discussion, showing empathy (that means picking your socks up off the bedroom floor, in case you were wondering). However, men, on the whole, show their love through physically doing something—earning money, cleaning the car, sexual contact. Sex, not discussion, is their way of showing love and feeling loved.

Men don't place enough value on emotional contact, and women don't place enough value on physical contact. That's fine when things are going well, as both partners "put out" for each other. But if a change happens in their lifestyle and one partner withdraws the contact the other needs, they get caught up in a vicious cycle. He isn't encouraged to extend emotional closeness to her while she's

Here's an idea for you... **Remember the old saying about walking in another's shoes if you want to understand them? When your partner has upset or irritated you, make a real effort to understand why they behaved in that way. Still confused? Make them explain what's going through their head. Silence is the worst thing you can do.**

withdrawing physical contact from him, and she in turn can't understand how he can expect her to have sex when they're barely grunting at each other and he spends entire evenings watching TV. Their sex life at best is mediocre, sporadic, and unsatisfying. And it stays that way.

This is the pattern of the sexually immature couple. They might have screwed like rabbits in their youth. They may have more sexual experience than Jack Nicholson and Russell Crowe combined. But sexual experience has nothing to do with sexual maturity.

SIGNS OF SEXUAL MATURITY

You don't wait for sex to just happen
You make sex a priority. You go to work when you're tired. You call your mother when you're stressed. You feed the kids when you have a headache. Sexually mature couples give sex the same priority they give other important things in their lives. They at least remain open to the idea of having sex at any time. They trust that their lover will find a way to turn them on.

You know the importance of doing it differently
Not least because your relationship, your body, and your life won't stay the same. Being prepared to change the way you have sex prepares you for the inevitable changes that will occur in your life. It's something that brings you respite when life

gets messy, joy when life gets dreary, and comfort when illness or death leave their scars on your psyche. Sex with your loving partner is where you go when you want to celebrate life's happiness, and it's where you run to hide from life's hurts.

Turn to IDEA 39, *Let a woman be a woman and a man be a man*, for ideas on finding new ways to relate to each other.

Try another idea...

You use sex as a way to show your partner that they're loved

Reaching out to your partner helps you avoid passive-aggressive games. You don't let just one person always initiate sex because that means the other has the power to refuse or withdraw. Sex can become a punishment or reward and if this is your relationship, that's a dangerous place to be, because both of you will end up hostile or resenting each other for different reasons.

You actively think of how you can use your sexuality to make your partner happier

This isn't just about giving your partner orgasms. Sex is a gift. You sometimes do stuff for no reward. Lots of people find it really difficult to make a gift of themselves. Even when they push themselves to sexual extremes in an effort to keep the spark between them alive, their relationship isn't intimate enough to maintain all the emotional intensity that scary sex throws up.

You try for each other

And by reading ideas like this you let the other person know it. Continually being prepared to go to bat for your relationship is as loving as it gets. Congratulations.

"The highest level of sexual excitement is in a monogamous relationship."
WARREN BEATTY, a man who should know

Defining idea...

How was
it for
you?

Q **The stuff about being intimate hit home. I feel that we're at our most awkward in bed. What should we do?**

A *This is really common. Was it always this way or did it happen after a big life change like having a baby? Sensate focus was invented for couples like you. Try in small ways to break down the barriers to intimacy and if you can't, couples counseling can help.*

Q **I get so angry with my partner. He puts little into our relationship and still expects sex. How can I deal with my resentment?**

A *Try having sex whenever he wants for a month. And initiate sex once a week. Break through your anger and hostility—and don't think I'm blaming you for being angry; it's just that it's not getting you anywhere. Show compassion. Show willingness. And if he's still expecting and not giving, insist that he spend half an hour talking to you every day. And if he won't do this, phone him. Relate.*

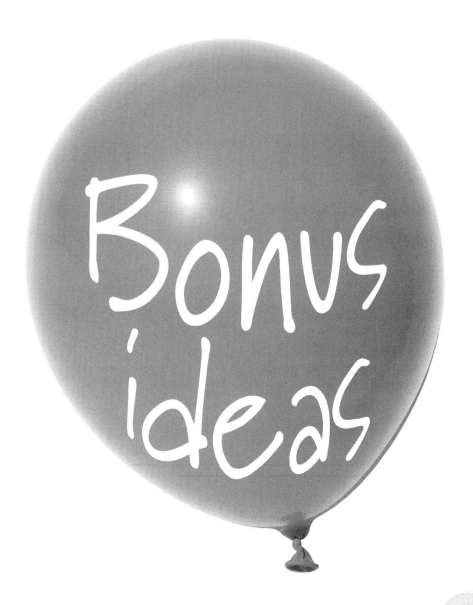

Bonus ideas

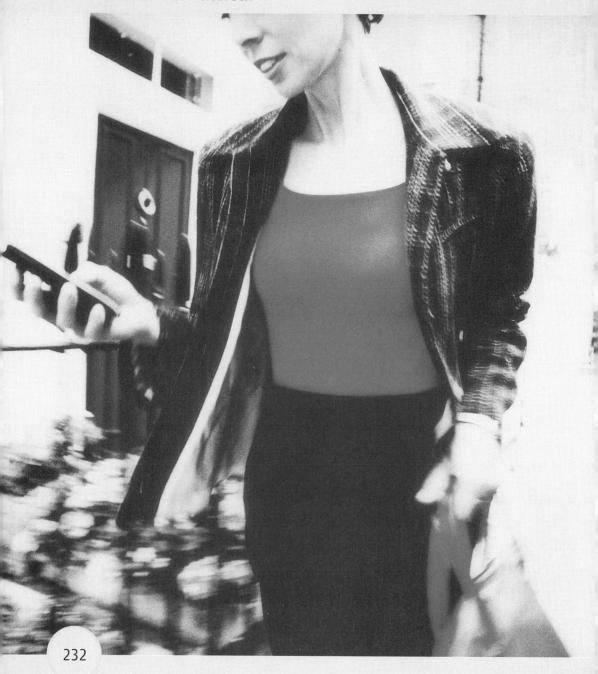

Pragma or manic?

Learning your lovestyle can help your love life, but not as much as learning your partner's lovestyle.

Knowing your own lovestyle helps you realize when you're making unrealistic demands of your lover. Knowing theirs is invaluable when they're getting on your nerves.

Psychologist John A. Lee interviewed hundreds of people and concluded that there were a number of different ways of "being" in a relationship. Understanding this makes it a whole lot easier to keep your sex life on course.

Lee's book *Lovestyles* can supply a definitive quiz to help you recognize you and your partner's lovestyle but this short version could give you some clues. Select the style or styles that seem more like you and your mate. According to Lee's research, 75 percent of the people in each group manifest these characteristics. Where do you fit in? (No one style is better than another, although clearly the styles that you're not are going to seem pretty damn weird.)

Are you eros?
- You see someone across a room and just "know" they're for you.
- Sexual feelings are important—love is central to your life.
- It's hard for you to find the right one—you're choosy.

Here's an idea for you...

Your lovestyle can vary depending on whom you're with— it's worthwhile thinking why you were, say, an erotic lover in one relationship but pragmatic in another. Are some characterisitcs helping or hindering your present relationship? Should you swap?

Are you ludus?

■ You hate to be tied down to events in the future with a partner.

■ In the past you have been accused of being emotionally immature or commitment-phobic.

■ You find loads of different types of people attractive.

Are you storge?

■ Love will fade but you can live with a friend for life.

■ Love is the basis of a strong community for you.

■ When you're good friends with someone, sexual problems can be resolved.

Are you mania?

■ To you being in love is synonymous with anxiety, even obsession.

■ You're capable of losing weight, sleep, and sometimes your sanity when you're truly in love.

■ It takes a long while for you to recover from a breakup— inevitably you're the dumped, not the dumper.

Are you pragma?

■ You have a shopping list of criteria that you expect your partner to fulfill.

■ You believe you can master any goal with common sense, including a succesful relationship.

■ You'd never end up with someone who didn't fit in with your ambitions for your life and your social group.

Eros lovers have an idealized physical image of their lover. But equally they believe they are on the planet to love one other person unstintingly—they've just got to find them! They stay loyal as long as romance is high on the agenda. If you're with an erotic lover, don't forget romance.

Still having trouble with communication? Try IDEA 20, *What's your LQ score?*

Try another idea...

Ludus lovers are often frustrated with aspects of their lives and are unwilling to commit themselves in a love relationship. A pure ludus will be concerned about causing hurt and warn lovers in advance that commitment is going to be shaky to put it mildly. Some are less scrupulous. Ludics avoid seeing the partner too often at the beginning of the relationship and even if they marry, there will often be distance and secrets. Love is a banquet and they want to try it all. This drives erotic and manic partners mad and their attitude bores and scares ludics.

Defining idea...

"A sour-grapes attitude, lingering feelings of hurt, or even the optimism of a new affair can cause you to rewrite the history of a past relationship. Some lovers, like those in the film *The Way We Were*, keep the good memories and forget the rest."
JOHN A. LEE, psychologist

Storge lovers often grow up in supportive families and communites. They expect lovers to be "special" friends. Storgics do not become preoccupied with love but in a long-term relationship they get very possessive if their love (their status quo) is threatened and will fight tooth and nail to retain their lover. If the commitment isn't there, sexual interest palls. Love is not an end in itself; it's part and parcel of their life or it doesn't work.

Mania lovers are the potential stalkers in the pack. They expect love to be dificult and all-absorbing and for them it is. They are jealous and possessive. It's a rare person who wants a long-term manic love and it's no surprise that they are almost inevitably abandoned.

Pragma lovers are the opposite. They don't fall in love with people who don't fit in with their lives, plans, and goals. They disdain excessive emotion and jealous scenes but they do appreciate signs of commitment. They'd like to have a love relationship but not if it means sacrificing peace of mind and their comfortable life. Most suited to living alone if it came to it, so beware if your partner is pragmatic—don't rock the boat too much.

How was it for you?

Q **I seem to be a mixture of Eros and Storge—can that be right?**

A *That would make you a Storgic Erotic. That's fine. One lovestyle often predominates but you can be a mixture of two or three. It's not worth getting hung up on this, it's not definitive. We are human after all. But it does help to make you more understanding of your partner's foibles.*

Q **How so?**

A *If you're with an erotic, just accept that they get horribly excited by visual images of people who fit into their ideal—which is why she's eyeing up the Italian waiter. But realizing that they are also the style who invest most in their romantic ideal of love may give you some reassurance. Similarly, if you're with a ludus, understanding that they are naturally restless may give you more patience with them. It's not just you—it's everything in their life that is vaguely dissatisfying. They can't help it—it's how they're made and you can't change it. Only they can.*

2

Slippery when wet

Different ways to get both your genitals glowing. Don't think prelude to penetration, savor it as the main event.

Play, touch, and intimacy are just as vital to foreplay as mastery of the basic sexual techniques. Tease each other and don't worry about going all the way.

There's no right way to do foreplay because everyone has a different sexual "script" of what turns them on, and what we feel like on Monday might not be the same thing we're in the mood for on Tuesday. The only way to indicate your preferences is to communicate, using your voice and body language—or even flaunting an established signal, such as wearing a particular dress or shade of lipstick that has become codified to indicate something naughty.

Ideally, touching and intimacy should be part of your relationship and not just restricted to the bedroom. Couples who are touchy-feely massage and cuddle each other while doing other things like watching TV and chatting to friends, and if you relish the touch of your lover at any time you're likely to move more quickly on to sexual play. Get your partner to be considerate to you in little things, like tidying up

Here's an idea for you...

Hang a sheet up in the middle of a room (or from a coat hanger on your closet door) and stand on either side of it so that you can't see each other. Naked, feel for each other through the sheet and rub lightly up against each other. What you think about during this, I'll leave to you. The novelty of the experience should make you feel aroused more quickly.

after himself; some psychologists think foreplay is the combined effect of your partner's behavior long before any sex takes place. Aline P. Zoldbrod says in *Sex Talk*: "There is something crucial before physical foreplay. It is all of the talking and actions that have happened during the last twelve hours or so of togetherness."

The secret to good foreplay is to stop seeing it as a prelude to intercourse. When we start a new relationship we spend a lot more time kissing, hugging, and touching, and we should be able to indulge in this at any time without needing to go all the way. Play around a little and find out what gets each other off. Get your partner to talk dirty to you, moan more, or indicate with their hands which spots feel good and, likewise, point him in the right direction. It could be that you just love having your toes sucked, your neck bitten, or your bottom spanked, but the only way to find out is to have lots of practice. It's actually more exciting if you get into the habit of playing around, with no pressure to reach orgasm or move on to penetrative sex; that way, each occasion keeps you both guessing. A lot of couples get into a kind of linear foreplay—first he feels your breasts, kisses you, and then moves down south, and after approximately five minutes you assume the missionary position. Sex doesn't have to be routine. Feel free to change the order in which you do things and to move from penetration to oral sex. Don't be afraid to lend a hand and play with yourself in front of him, too.

Defining idea...

"Too much of a good thing is wonderful."
MAE WEST

On average we devote around twenty minutes to foreplay, according to the Durex 2004 Global Sex Survey. If your partner rushes things, play around while you are still fully clothed. Rubbing yourself against his hard crotch through your jeans can feel magnificent, and when he touches your naked body it'll feel

"The sexual embrace can only be compared with music and with prayer."
HAVELOCK ELLIS, author and researcher

Defining idea...

better if you're already hot. Before you get to naked genital contact, try kissing, light touches (with fingertips or feathers), and breast and neck play. He could try cupping your genitals with one hand while the other presses on your pubic bone. If you like oral sex, try it in different positions; for instance, receiving it while in the doggy position feels completely different from lying on your back. If your partner is licking/kissing you, he can also try varying from hot/cold temperatures or sucking a mint or cough lozenge, all of which will change how his tongue feels.

Play around a little and don't be afraid to introduce sex toys. Whatever you do, keep it fun and sexy. You know what they say, sometimes it's more fun to travel than to arrive!

How was it for you?

Q How long should it take for me to get aroused during foreplay?

A *There is no set time, although Dr. Ian Kerner says in his book* She Comes First *that if their partner spends at least twenty-one minutes on foreplay, 92.3 percent of women are guaranteed an orgasm. His results, though, are based on a small sample. Other women need much more or less than this. Women over thirty-five tend to prefer less foreplay, whereas men of the same age are likely to want more (men need more stimulation as they get older to maintain an erection). Many women complain they don't get enough foreplay, but it could be that their partners are doing what they think turns them on and not what actually does. Tell him what you want. To slow him down, find non-genital ways of stimulating him, such as rubbing his perineum or massaging his stomach.*

Q Why do men get aroused so much more quickly than women?

A *Perhaps because a penis is so much more of a hands-on piece of anatomy. A man knows he's aroused when his penis is hard, but often women have no physical clue. Having a wet pussy doesn't mean you're aroused, as vaginal lubrication depends on where you are in your cycle and what medications you're taking. Researchers have also found that a lot of foreplay is led by the male partners, so use a bit of girl power!*

This idea originally appeared in *Incredible Orgasms*, by Marcelle Perks.

3

Vital energy

We need an endless supply of energy to do everything we need and want to do in our lives, yet we're often overwhelmed by a desire to have a swift forty winks.

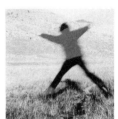

Have you ever felt like curling up under your desk and spending the afternoon snoozing? Or been in serious need of matchsticks to prop your eyelids open? And do you ever wonder why this always seems to happen in the middle of a vital meeting, despite three cups of coffee?

THE ENERGY EQUATION

We need sugar (glucose) to fire our system. It's the fuel that gives us our energy. However, too much is deemed by our body to be dangerous (think of diabetics).

We obtain this fuel largely from our food. A hormone called insulin specifically lowers these blood sugar levels and adjusts them according to our minute-by-minute

Get a good breakfast in! A recent study revealed that people who didn't eat breakfast were likely to be overweight and less intelligent. So, if you didn't have a good reason before, you do now. A good breakfast will sustain you through to lunch, but remember that sugary cereals will pick you up and then drop you like a stone.

needs. We don't have very much sugar circulating at any one time because as soon as we do, in comes insulin to normalize the level. When blood sugar levels are low, we rely on stored glucose (glycogen) found in the muscles and the liver, which helps maintain this delicate equilibrium. Once stored glucose is used, more food will be required to sustain glucose production.

Not all food was created equal. Some foods "burn" (meaning they're converted into sugar) quickly while other foods "burn" slowly. These foods are called low and high glycemic index foods (GI foods). The GI index is a way of measuring foods that are converted to glucose at different rates. But don't get hung up on the GI index, as confusingly you'll see it published in different places with different values. As a very simple rule of thumb, white things (e.g., potatoes, pasta, bread, parsnips, white rice) are like rocket fuel, while dense, thick, fibrous brown or green things (e.g., lentils, chickpeas, broccoli, brown rice) are going to burn more slowly and are our great energy sustainers. For example, whereas glucose (sugar) scores 100 on the GI scale, a lentil comes in at a cool 42. The important thing to remember is that it isn't necessarily foods that we traditionally think of as sweet that cause the problems. A sweet potato, for instance, actually scores quite low, as it is wonderfully fibrous.

You can raise your blood sugar by another mechanism. Stick your head in the mouth of a man-eating shark, then quickly take it out again and swim like hell for the shore. This would certainly pick your blood sugar up rapidly, as powerful stress hormones would raise blood sugar to give you enough energy for your clever exit strategy. We do this all the time, but usually our boss, gas bill, or deadline is the cause of our stress and not man-eating sharks. Of course, there is an easier way of picking up blood sugar levels—have a cigarette or a cup of coffee. These are both stimulants, which stimulate the adrenal glands (where those stress hormones come from) to release sugar from storage. But what goes up, must come down, hence staying awake in the meeting becomes a challenge.

So, what's the problem with the blood sugar whizzing up and down all the time? First, the pancreas, where all that insulin is produced, is going to get worn out. Second, you're going to get dips of energy as the blood sugar levels plummet when insulin tries to lower them. Third, insulin is also a fat storage hormone, so if it overreacts and there's continuously too much insulin in the system, eventually you'll put on weight. Commonly, this appears as those cute love handles or that attractive tire around the middle. And where do you see this phenomena most commonly? On stressed-out executives who are eating the wrong things, having too many cups of coffee, and getting stressed-out.

Defining idea...

"Mary: I want a guy who can play 36 holes of golf, and still have enough energy to take Warren and me to a baseball game, and eat sausages, and beer, not light beer, but beer. That's my ad, print it up. Brenda: 'Fatty who likes golf, beer, and baseball.' Gee, Mary, where are you gonna find a gem like that?"
THERE'S SOMETHING ABOUT MARY, a lesson in why you should be careful how you define "energy"

How was
it for
you?

Q   I'm starving by 11:00 a.m. How do I avoid stuffing my face with chocolate?

A   *Make sure you really are getting a good breakfast. By that I mean one with a low GI score. Good foods for breakfast include eggs with rye toast, sardines on toast, yogurt with ground nuts and seeds, and oats with fruits, nuts, and seeds.*

Q   What if I don't have the time for cooking?

A   *Making breakfast is really quick once you get organized and get the right foods in. Unless you're very on the ball, you might not want to bring your lunch into work in a Tupperware container. You might have to find lunch on the hoof. Although a baked potato has a high GI score, a little protein brings it down, so add some cottage cheese or tuna. Dinner is easy to organize—steam some vegetables and grill some fish or chicken. Start looking at recipe books for inspiration—you don't actually have to follow them to the letter. Once you're used to cooking, it really is quicker than opening a package or can.*

Q   What if I don't have the time to go shopping?

A   *Have you tried shopping online? Once it's set up it's wonderfully easy. Sites that promise hour delivery slots are best; otherwise you have to hang around for them to deliver, which is a pain. The key phrase is, "Be prepared."*

This idea originally appeared in *Boost Your Whole Health*, by Kate Cook.

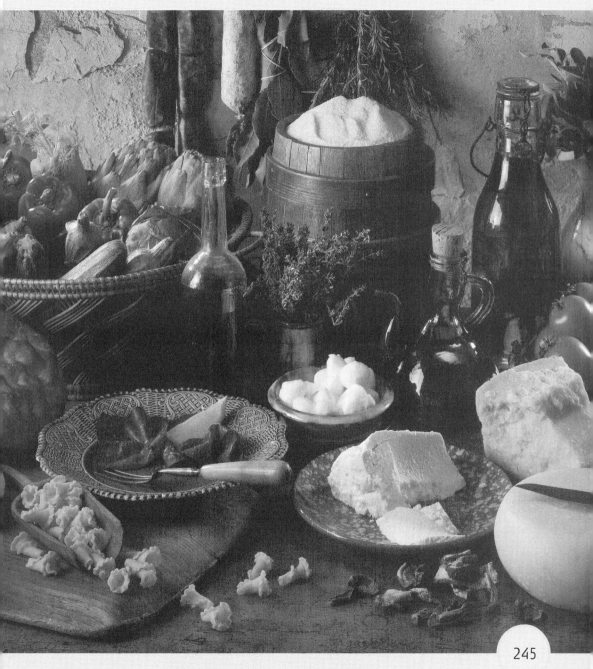

Where it's at...

52 Brilliant Ideas

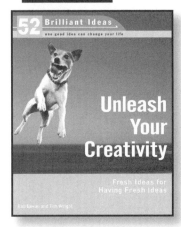

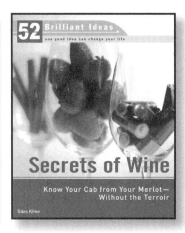

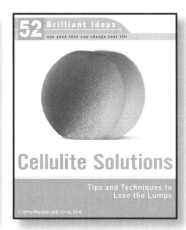

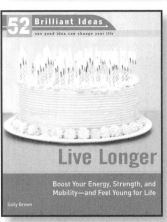

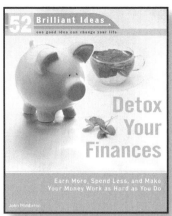

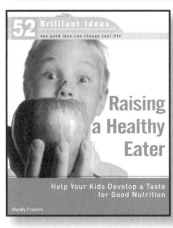

UNLEASH YOUR CREATIVITY
978-0-399-53325-9

LIVE LONGER
978-0-399-53302-0

SECRETS OF WINE
978-0-399-53348-8

DETOX YOUR FINANCES
978-0-399-53301-3

CELLULITE SOLUTIONS
978-0-399-53326-6

RAISING A HEALTHY EATER
978-0-399-53339-6

PERIGEE   An imprint of Penguin Group (USA)

one good idea can change your life

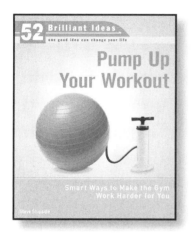
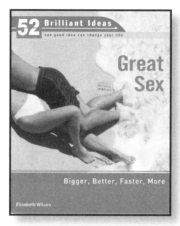
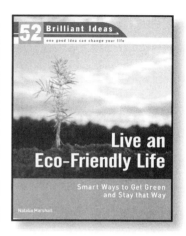
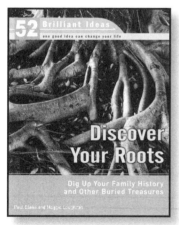
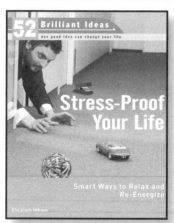
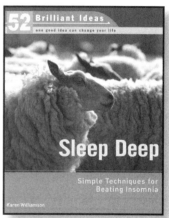

PUMP UP YOUR WORKOUT
978-0-399-53409-6

GREAT SEX
978-0-399-53392-1

**LIVE AN ECO-
FRIENDLY LIFE**
978-0-399-53396-9

DISCOVER YOUR ROOTS
978-0-399-53322-8

**STRESS-PROOF
YOUR LIFE**
978-0-399-53405-8

SLEEP DEEP
978-0-399-53323-5

Available wherever books are sold or at penguin.com